Families, Physicians, and Children with Special Health Needs

Families, Physicians, and Children with Special Health Needs

COLLABORATIVE MEDICAL EDUCATION MODELS

EDITED BY
Rosalyn Benjamin Darling
and Margo I. Peter

FOREWORD BY
Merle McPherson and Bonnie Strickland

An Exceptional Parent Press Publication

AUBURN HOUSE
Westport, Connecticut • London

Library of Congress Cataloging-in-Publication Data

Families, physicians, and children with special health needs :
collaborative medical education models / edited by Rosalyn Benjamin
Darling and Margo I. Peter ; foreword by Merle McPherson and Bonnie
Strickland.
p. cm.
"An Exceptional Parent Press publication".
Includes bibliographical references and index.
ISBN 0–86569–226–2 (alk. paper)
1. Community health services for children—United States.
2. Pediatrics—Study and teaching—United States. 3. Exceptional
children—Medical care—United States. 4. Handicapped children—
Medical care—United States. I. Darling, Rosalyn Benjamin.
II. Peter, Margo I.
RJ102.F36 1994
362.1'9892'000973—dc20 93–40559

British Library Cataloguing in Publication Data is available.

Library of Congress Catalog Card Number: 93–40559
ISBN: 0–86569–226–2

First published in 1994

Auburn House, 88 Post Road West, Westport, CT 06881
An imprint of Greenwood Publishing Group, Inc.

Printed in the United States of America

The paper used in this book complies with the
Permanent Paper Standard issued by the National
Information Standards Organization (Z39.48–1984).

10 9 8 7 6 5 4 3 2 1

Copyright Acknowledgments

The editors and publisher gratefully acknowledge permission for use of the following material:

From R. B. Darling, "Parent–Professional Interaction: The Roots of Misunderstanding," in M. Seligman, ed., *The Family with a Handicapped Child*, 2nd ed., 1991. Used with permission of Allyn & Bacon.

From S. D. Klein, "The Role of the Family in Helping the Child with Learning Disabilities," in M. Davis and J. C. Whitener, *The Role of Vision in Multidisciplinary Approaches to Children with Learning Disabilities*, 1981. Courtesy of Charles C Thomas, Publisher, Springfield, Illinois.

From S. D. Klein and R. E. Klein, "Delivering Bad News: The Most Challenging Task in Patient Education," in *Journal of the American Optometric Association* 9 (1987): 660–663.

From R. B. Darling, *Families Against Society: A Study of Reactions to Children with Birth Defects*, 1979. Used with permission of Sage Publications.

To our families, and especially to

Eric and Susan as they prepare to add a new branch to our family tree—R. B. D.

Dr. James Bibb and Ila Peter, who have taught me about family centered care just by being my family—M. I. P.

Contents

Foreword
Merle McPherson and Bonnie Strickland ix

Preface xv

1 Introduction: The Need to Teach the Family's Perspective to Physicians
Rosalyn Benjamin Darling 1

Part I The Family's Perspective

2 Collaboration Defined Mathematically
Florene Stewart Poyadue 17

3 The Miracle of Michael
Sharon L. Spano 29

4 The Challenge of Communication with Parents
Stanley D. Klein 51

Part II Models of Health Provider Education

Preservice Models

5 A First-year Medical Student Curriculum about Family Views of Chronic and Disabling Conditions
Judy Lewis and Robert M. Greenstein 77

6 Parents as Educators of Medical Students
Nancy J. DiVenere 101

7 Graduate Medical Education in Pediatrics: Preparing Reliable Allies for Parents of Children with Special Health Care Needs
W. Carl Cooley 109

Continuing Education Models

8 Preparing Physicians through Continuing Medical Education
Margo I. Peter and Calvin C. J. Sia 123

9 Overcoming Obstacles to Early Intervention Referral: The Development of a Video-based Training Model for Community Physicians
Rosalyn Benjamin Darling 135

10 What Do Physicians Want to Know? A Statewide Survey Report of Physicians' Needs for Information about Early Intervention
Francine Gortler Gallagher and Corinne W. Garland 149

Part III Directions in Medical Education and Family-centered Care: Prospects for the 1990s and Beyond

11 Health Care for Children with Disabilities: A Contemporary View
Alfred Healy 173

12 Conclusion: Building on Existing Models to Expand Training Opportunities in the Future
Margo I. Peter and Rosalyn Benjamin Darling 185

Resource List 191

Index 195

About the Editors and Contributors 201

Foreword

Merle McPherson
and
Bonnie Strickland

As we draw closer to a national health care program for all Americans, many issues have emerged that are related to the care of children with special health care needs—and to their caretaking families. Such issues emphasize the many common needs of all children and families, as well as the unique needs of specific populations including children with a variety of actual and potentially disabling conditions such as cerebral palsy, Down syndrome, asthma, diabetes, HIV/AIDS, emotional disorders, hemophilia, genetic disorders, and health-related educational and behavioral problems. Increased numbers of currently uninsured or uninsurable children (e.g., those with "preexisting condition" exclusions) will be covered. Portability of health coverage will allow families choices in jobs without fear of lost insurance coverage. Primary care providers will gain increased responsibility through managed care referrals, review arrangements (gatekeeper), and reimbursement incentives. Specialty providers will benefit from alliances with primary care providers. Families, however, may face gaps in covered benefits for children with significant special health care needs, and access to the highest cost specialty services may be restricted in capitated systems. Learning to work together with a wide range of providers, both at the community level and in tertiary centers, will be critical in overcoming these barriers. Medical education programs must play a critical role in assuring that physicians have the needed skills and knowledge to practice in the new system.

As availability of care becomes a reality, we must also insure the accessibility and quality of that care. While health care reform has many training implications in regard to the availability and comprehensiveness of health care, another more subtle national movement has been under way, which deals not so much with health care services themselves as with the context in which health and other community services are developed, coordinated, and provided to children and families living in the nation's communities. This initiative, legislated by OBRA 1989 and supported by health, education, mental health, and social service agencies at the federal level, is an attempt to reframe, or reinvent, the context in which services are provided to children with special health care needs and their families. "Community-based systems of care," as this initiative is referred to, is based on the concept that all services, including health care, must be systematically developed, linked, and coordinated at the community level in a way that assures the needs of children and families are addressed in a family-centered and culturally competent manner. The principles of the community-based system have been specifically defined, and form the basis of a national priority for providing care to children with special health care needs and their families. The elements of this system include the following:

- Service to a broad population of children with special health care needs who have health problems requiring something beyond routine and basic care;
- Comprehensive services that are available and accessible for both children with special health care needs and their families;
- Provision of needed services to children with special health care needs and their families in or near their home communities, to the extent possible;
- Provision of services from different providers in a complementary and consistent manner; and
- Provision of services that are family centered.

These principles of family-centered, community-based systems of care will undoubtedly provide the context in which the nation's health policy will be implemented. Because this framework will significantly influence service delivery, it provides both a timely incentive and an exciting opportunity for examining and restructuring models of medical education from a systems-oriented perspective.

What must be included in a medical education model that emphasizes community-based systems of care? And how does it differ from a more traditional model? First, while the newer systems-based models retain the state-of-the-art clinical-specific emphasis of their more traditional counterparts, attention is also given to the context, or framework, in which discipline-specific skills are practiced. For example, within a community-based system, care is provided within the context of the family, and the system is designed to be responsive to family needs. Traditional models of medical education may focus primarily, and sometimes solely, on acquisition of specific clinical skills and information, with lesser emphasis on how to apply newly acquired skills within the framework of family-centered care. In a systems-oriented model, training is specifically designed not only to ensure the acquisition of clinical information, but also to address issues related to the impact on the family. Thus, while acquiring and updating technical knowledge, the physician might also learn—perhaps from families—the cultural implications and family issues associated with specific health and medical procedures; information on the emotional and financial support needed by families; and the strengths of families in providing continuity in the care of their child. Technical training, provided in the context of family-centered care, provides a model for how—not necessarily what—services are provided. The element of family-centered care is one essential element of a systems-oriented approach to training, and one that provides the major emphasis of this book.

Second, a systems-oriented training model redefines and broadens the role of the physician (and all other providers) within the context of the "system" of care, rather than as an independent entity. This broader role gives the physician the responsibility for ensuring that services for a child and family are coordinated, complementary, and consistent among providers. Physicians, for example, represent only one component of the community-based system that addresses the comprehensive needs of families. Physicians—as well as education, social services, and other health care providers—must, in a community-based system of care, assume broader roles that bridge the gap between the multitude of services provided to a single child and family. When operationalized, this means that systems-oriented training models place substantial emphasis on the role of the health professional in cooperative planning and communication within and outside the health profession, active coordination of services, and community planning activities on behalf of the children and families they serve. Thus, some part of training must be interprofessional and address health issues as they interrelate with other aspects of the service community.

Third, a systems-oriented medical education program emphasizes the community as the focal point for creating, delivering, and ensuring the quality of services provided to children with special needs and their families. Maximizing the availability of care within the child's home community requires families and providers to challenge some aspects of traditional service models and to develop and implement new alternatives for children and families. One such alternative has been the development of the "medical home" concept, which assures every child of a single and personal source of health care in the community, and at the same time provides referral to and coordination with other service providers. The familiarity and coordination that characterize this model encourage the development of community-based support, which can reduce the need for extended hospitalization and frequent long-distance travel. Although this concept is the embodiment of a community-based systems approach to health care, not all physicians have the skills to make the medical home a reality. Medical education programs must assume responsibility for preparing physicians for this new role.

Fourth, medical education models that emphasize community-based systems of services can also be distinguished in the way in which the content of the training program is developed. Developing innovative—not just new—models of medical education based on the community system creates a challenge for those responsible for preservice and continuing education programs. Innovative models are those that are receptive and responsive to the changing needs of the nation, and truly responsive to the identified needs of the communities they are intended to serve. Just as the principles of family-centered care begin with families at the community level and then evolve to influence and form the basis of a national policy of family-centered care, so too must models of medical education also stem from identification of the best practices within real community settings, be translated into operational principles, and then be incorporated into the medical schools and teaching hospitals.

Fifth, because communities and the systems of care that characterize them are changing continuously, medical education programs must remain flexible and responsive to issues that create or promote changes in the way services are provided. Rigid, unchanging, programmatic structures lack the dynamic elements so essential for systems-based education models. Too often, in traditional program models, little relationship exists between the content of the training program and the real needs of communities in which families live and professionals practice. To avoid this, training programs must ensure an ongoing mechanism for listening to families and community-based physicians and for including community-related systems issues in the training program. Community surveys, consumer focus groups, and identification of actual programs that exemplify the principles of best practice in regard to systems development are only a few examples of how the community can serve to inform and enrich the content of medical education programs.

Sixth and finally, medical education programs must assume responsibility for creating a more integrated community-based system of services through leadership training. How to produce physician leaders responsive to the changing needs of communities is an ongoing, but now urgent, agenda, as the traditional roles of service providers change in response to the national health agenda. Systems change, in itself, is not a new topic, and we know that sustainable change requires strong commitment and incentive at every level. We know that simply adding requirements to already overcrowded medical school and residency programs does not produce professionals who know how to work within coordinated systems of community-based care. Training programs may have to be completely redesigned, emphasizing what we know is critical to the development of the skills we want professionals to have. For example, to develop future physician leaders who can view health issues from a broad, interprofessional perspective, medical education programs must offer physicians opportunities for extended exposure to real community issues related to, but perhaps outside, their own specific areas of clinical expertise.

In summary, there is no question that health care reform will require a significant departure from traditional models of care. And there is no doubt that the community-based system will provide the context for providing health care for all children and families, including those with special needs. Medical education programs must accept the challenge of incorporating what we have learned about the characteristics of quality systems of care into dynamic training models, clearly based on the established best practices of comprehensive, community-based, family-centered care. We know the same level of medical skills and knowledge will be expected of physicians as is expected in more traditional models of health care. What must change is the knowledge and skills with which the provider approaches and interacts with the community itself, other providers, and—most importantly—the children and families served by the system.

This book provides models that embody the principles and practices characterizing a family-centered system of community-based health care for families and children. Throughout the text, the principles of best practice in community-based health care are operationalized and defined in thoughtful, family-centered terms that clearly reflect their community orientation. The models presented provide a qualitative companion to health care reform and provide an opportunity for renewing and enriching the framework within which we prepare physicians to serve our most valuable commodities: the children and families of our nation's communities.

Preface

This book is being published at an exciting time in the history of medical care. Universal health insurance is on the nation's agenda; in the near future, all children may have access to the care they need. Yet, the path that this care will follow is still uncertain. Individuals and groups concerned with family-centered care are wondering how concepts like managed care will interface with a perspective that values the family's priorities and concerns as much as those of care providers or funders. Policymakers must face the challenge of reconciling recent family-centered public policies with the imperatives of fiscal restraint. Some of the material in this book may be helpful in future discussions about health care priorities. Certainly, the chapter authors make a convincing case for not overlooking the "human" side of medicine. We are indebted to them for this contribution.

A number of people were instrumental in bringing about the publication of this book. We would like to thank Stanley Klein for first suggesting that the book be written. His encouragement and aid began the publication process. Carl Cooley provided valuable assistance, both in collecting information from various sources and in contacting potential prepublication reviewers. We would like to thank Suzanne Yunghans at the Pennsylvania Chapter of the American Academy of Pediatrics and Cindy Gossard at Beginnings for their assistance in organizing the conference on which this book was based. Also, Anne Ambrose at the Hawaii Medical Association spent many hours transcribing the conference proceedings, which provided the basis for several of the book's chapters. Finally, we would like to thank our editors at Greenwood for facilitating the publication process.

Rosalyn Benjamin Darling would like to thank the staff at Beginnings, whose dedication and skill made it possible to take the time to edit this volume. Thanks also to Jon, who was, as always, a source of support and assistance, and to Seth, who graciously and competently accepted the responsibilities that came with being the child of busy parents.

Margo Peter would like to thank the staff of the Medical Home Project, who worked so hard to implement a vision of CME training programs for physicians in Hawaii. Mahalo to Sharon Taba, Alix Howard-Jones and Anne Ambrose for their persistent efforts. Thanks also go to Dr. Nancy Kuntz and Susan Rocco who "walked the talk" of family-centered care and worked so effectively as a training team for the project. The support and encouragement provided by Dr. Merle McPherson were invaluable, and she deserves special recognition for her efforts to promote family-centered care. A very special thank you to Dr. Calvin Sia; his efforts on behalf of children are a constant inspiration, and his vision has been a guiding light.

We both would like to thank all of the families with whom we have worked over the years. They have inspired us and taught us the value of family-centered care. We hope that this book will add in some small way to the quality of their lives and the lives of other families with children who have special health needs in the years to come.

Families, Physicians, and Children with Special Health Needs

1

Introduction: The Need to Teach the Family's Perspective to Physicians

Rosalyn Benjamin Darling

Interactions between families and the professionals who serve them have often been strained. Families of children with special health needs, especially, have noted difficulties in their communications with physicians and other medical professionals. Betty Pieper, the parent of a child with disabilities and an advocate for families, has written,

> I have heard the stories of hundreds of parents. . . . With rare exceptions they are all the same in essence. . . . The pain, frustration, and anxiety of professionals result in curtness to the point of rudeness, technical jargon to the point of insensibility, and other well-known behaviors that aid them in distancing themselves from us just when we need human contact the most. (in Darling & Darling, 1982, p. vii)

The two interactional areas that seem to be most problematic are those of diagnosis, or providing the first information to families about a child's disability, and ongoing primary care—both routine and in the case of acute illness—for the child with a chronic health condition or disability. A number of studies (see, e.g., Claflin & Meisels, 1993) have reported that parents of high-risk, chronically ill, and disabled infants continue to recall interactions with health care providers as one of the most stressful parts of their early experiences with their children. (See Darling, 1979, for numerous examples of negative parent–physician encounters.)

Although the literature is replete with examples of interactional difficulties of this kind, a promising trend has become apparent in recent years.

Initiatives by both parents and professionals have led to physician education models that have taught concepts such as "family-centered care." These models can now be found in medical school and residency curricula and in continuing education programs for community physicians. In 1991, the editors of this volume discussed the need for the developers and users of these models to share and coordinate their efforts. As a result, they organized, along with Sheila Cannon (a parent) and Drs. W. Carl Cooley and Alan Kohrt (both pediatricians), a national conference entitled "Creating Family–Professional Partnerships: Educating Physicians and Other Health Professionals to Care for Children with Chronic and Disabling Conditions." That conference led to this book.

The conference, which was held in Pittsburgh in May 1992, was sponsored by Beginnings Early Intervention Services of Cambria County, the Pennsylvania Chapter of the American Academy of Pediatrics, and Project Caring, with support from the Pennsylvania Department of Public Welfare, the U.S. Maternal and Child Health Bureau, the Pennsylvania Developmental Disabilities Planning Council, the Medical Home Project of the Hawaii Medical Association, and the Parent–Professional Partnership of Children's Hospital–Pittsburgh. The conference brought together more than one hundred parents and professionals from twenty-five states, who shared their experiences during two days of presentations and discussions. Presenters representing a diversity of approaches to medical education were invited to write chapters for this book. The models and viewpoints represented include those of physicians, early intervention professionals, professionals with backgrounds in education, psychology, and sociology, and parents.

This chapter will provide an overview of some of the difficulties faced by physicians and families of children with special health needs in their interactions with one another, as well as a summary of the trend away from older clinical approaches toward more family-centered care. All of the other chapters will reflect this trend in their emphasis on teaching the family's perspective to physicians.

FAMILY–PHYSICIAN INTERACTION[1]

Worldviews and Their Sources

Sociologists use the concept of worldview to describe the way individuals and groups perceive and define the events they encounter in everyday life. Members of the same cultural group tend to have similar worldviews.

However, to the extent that their life experiences differ, individuals may have views that diverge markedly from those of others. Because their life experiences and consequent expectations differ, parents and professionals often approach children with disabilities from different perspectives. As a result, parent–professional interactions are strained, and conflict is a common outcome. As Freidson wrote, "the separate worlds of experience and reference of the layman and the professional worker are always in potential conflict with each other" (1961, p. 175).

Knowledge, beliefs, attitudes, and opinions about a subject are learned through experience—at home, at school, on the job. Many parents have little knowledge of children before they have children of their own. The parenting experience is a powerful means of socialization that shapes parents' views of child development and appropriate parental behavior. Similarly, physicians and other professionals acquire their views from their educational training and subsequent professional experience, as well as from their day-to-day experiences. A professional who is not a parent cannot understand parenthood from the same perspective that the parent of five children has. Similarly, a parent of a typical child cannot understand the experience of parenting a child with a disability in the same way as the disabled child's parent. As the mother of a child with spina bifida explained,

> The doctor says "Don't put her in diapers," and comes down hard on me when I do. . . . The last time I tried [putting her in panties], we both ended up being embarrassed in public. . . . Medical professionals see things only one way. They have no idea how the problem affects the family. (Spina Bifida Association of America, 1982)

In one study (Wolraich, 1980), a majority of pediatric practitioners reported no nonprofessional contact with developmentally disabled individuals; in another small sample of pediatricians (Darling, 1979), less than 7 percent had an immediate family member who had a disability.

The opposing worldviews of parents and professionals can be summarized by a typology suggested by Parsons (1951). According to Parsons, the role of the professional in our society is characterized by the traits of achievement, universalism, functional specificity, and affective neutrality. When the Parsonian typology is applied to parents of children with disabilities, their role can be characterized by the traits of ascription, particularism, functional diffuseness, and affectivity. In addition, the professional role is marked by dominance, and the parent role is marked

Table 1–1
Ideal-typical Role Patterns of Professionals and Parents

Professional	Parent
Achieved	Ascribed
Universalistic	Particularistic
Functionally specific	Functionally diffuse
Affectively neutral	Affective
Dominant	Anomic

Source: Parsons (1951).

by anomie and submission (see Table 1–1). Although these are ideal-typical traits that do not always apply to individual professionals or parents, they describe the normative expectations that accompany the parent and professional *roles* in American society today.

Achievement/Ascription

Whereas the status of the professional is *achieved*, the status of the parent of a child with a disability is *ascribed*. In other words, because professionals *choose* their careers, they are likely to expect the freedom to practice in a manner that is interesting and rewarding to them. As a result, many do not want to be "bothered" with the problems of disabled children. Parents, on the other hand, have little choice; they have given birth to a child with a chronic problem, whose care they are expected to assume. Although parenthood is an "achieved" status, if given a choice, virtually no parents would want their children to have disabilities. Most, however, come to love their children and to accept society's expectations about good parenting and doing everything possible to help their children develop to their fullest potential. These parents become frustrated when they interact with professionals who do not share their parental enthusiasm. They may also come to resent the professional who deals with their problems during working hours, whereas they deal with them twenty-four hours a day.

Universalism/Particularism

The professional is concerned with all cases of a particular type, and the parents are concerned with only one case: their own child. The universalistic orientation of the professional is reflected in the bureaucratic structure of clinical practice and the tendency to treat all patients in a like manner, regardless of each patient's unique personal situation.

Professionals tend to categorize their patients on the basis of clinical theory and past personal and clinical experience. Resulting generalizations may lead professionals to make inappropriate assumptions about children with disabilities or their parents. For example, professionals have tended to overestimate the negative impact on the family of a child with a disability (Blackard & Barsch, 1984; Sloper & Turner, 1991). Pieper (in Darling & Darling, 1982) noted anecdotally a case in which a professional gave parents a long lecture about their guilt over having given birth to a disabled child, only to learn that the child who was the subject of their discussion was adopted.

Parents resent universalistic treatment. For them, *this* child is important. Parental reports like the following are illustrative.

> Whenever there's something wrong, our pediatrician says, "I don't know what I can do for you. That's her condition." . . . He blames all of her [medical] problems on retardation instead of treating them.
>
> —mother of a child with severe mental retardation
>
> She had a problem with her knee, and we took her to Children's Hospital. . . . They said, "There's nothing we can do with one of *these* children."
>
> —father of a child with Down syndrome
>
> [Our pediatrician] treated her as an article in a medical journal.
>
> —mother of a child with a rare congenital syndrome

(all in Darling, 1979, pp. 151, 152)

Specificity/Diffuseness

As Mercer (1965) noted, families may be regarded from either a clinical or a social system perspective. In the clinical perspective, the family is defined in terms of their "problem"; in the social system perspective, all of the family's roles—in addition to the role of "family with a problem"—are taken into account. Most medical professionals have traditionally employed a clinical perspective, in which the presenting problem or symptoms become paramount and other roles played by the patient in the community are ignored. Thus the hospital patient becomes "the gall bladder in Room 23," even though he is also a husband, a father, a carpenter, and a churchgoer. One adult with cerebral palsy noted that the message constantly communicated by professionals was, "Your weakest point is what is most important to us, we don't care about the rest of you" (Richardson, 1972, p. 533). Similarly, the father of a child with mental retardation and cerebral palsy remarked, "The pediatrician . . . wasn't interested in Brian as a *person*" (Darling, 1979, p. 152).

Parents see their children playing a variety of social roles: loving son or daughter, sibling, grandchild, playmate, and student, as well as child with a disability. Their relationship to their child is *diffuse*, involving all of these roles. Sometimes, when a child's disability does not conflict with the roles played by the child in a family setting, parents do not define the child as disabled at all. A child with a learning disability, for example, may be regarded as nondisabled at home and in the neighborhood. The parents of such a child may resent a label applied by professional educators that is not relevant to their experience. Professionals sometimes accuse such parents of denying reality; their unidimensional perspective prevents them from realizing that the parents' "reality" may be very different from their own.

Affective Neutrality/Affectivity

In their training, professionals are often cautioned about becoming too emotionally involved with the families they serve. Overinvolvement is believed to impair the professional's ability to provide effective treatment. Consequently, many professionals seek to maintain some emotional distance between themselves and their patients or clients. Stacey (1980) and others have noted, further, that professionals are often not trained in techniques of counseling or supportive communication.

On the other hand, studies have shown that patients generally expect their physicians to satisfy their socioemotional needs. Freidson (1961) found that patients expected their physicians to be *both* technically competent and able to satisfy emotional needs. Another study (Hickson, Altemeier & O'Connor, 1983) found that, although only 30 percent of the mothers seeking care in private pediatric offices were most concerned about their children's physical health, most parent–physician communication involved only this topic. Psychosocial concerns were not raised because parents believed that pediatricians were not interested in helping them in that area. Pediatricians, on the other hand, assumed that parents were not interested in discussing their psychosocial concerns with them. Many parents interpret professionals' affective neutrality to mean that these professionals do not care about their children.

Professional Dominance/Anomie

The sociological concept that best characterizes the situation of many families when they first learn or suspect that their child has a serious problem is *anomie*. Anomie involves either meaninglessness or powerlessness or both. When physicians fail to provide clear diagnostic and prognostic information, parents typically embark on a search for answers.

Most parents believe that they cannot help their child until they have defined their situation. Research (see, e.g., Seligman & Darling, 1989) has shown that the need for information is the greatest need these parents have, early in their children's lives. Even after their need for meaning has been met, parents may continue to feel powerless, however.

Generally, both professionals and parents have a need to be in control of their situations of mutual interaction. Typically, as Freidson (1970) and others have shown, professionals retain control. The ritualized routine of clinical practice supports the professional's dominance. Parents, on the other hand, are likely to feel powerless and resent the professional's control over their lives.

Parents usually do not openly challenge professional dominance, however. As Strong noted in a study of two hospital outpatient departments, "Many parents disagreed strongly with the doctors' verdict at one time or another. Nevertheless all but a handful made no direct challenge to their authority. Most maintained an outward pose of agreement with what they were told" (1979, p. 87). Stimson and Webb explained patients' reticence to challenge the physician as follows:

> Our observations and interviews lead us to suggest that the doctor is aided in his ability to exert control over the information he gives and in his way of acting towards patients by their desire to please him, to emerge from the encounter without loss of face. (Stimson & Webb, 1975, p. 127)

Parents *do* often complain about professionals after they have left the clinical setting. Parents' support groups serve an important function by providing a forum for storytelling. As a result of interaction in such groups, many parents change physicians or explore alternative treatment modes against the advice of professionals. As Stimson and Webb noted, "Whilst the patient's ability to control the outcome of the consultation is limited, he has considerable ability to control what happens after he has left the doctor's presence" (1975, p. 87). Noncompliance with professional advice appears to be related, at least in part, to lack of satisfaction during the parent–professional encounter. Francis, Korsch, and Morris (1968) found in a study of outpatient visits to a children's hospital that the extent to which parents' expectations were not met, lack of warmth in the physician–parent relationship, and failure to receive a diagnostic explanation were the key factors in noncompliance. Parents who do not have access to supportive interactions outside of the clinical setting may continue to feel powerless in the face of professional dominance.

New Directions in Professional Training and Parent Activism

Are the worldviews of parents and professionals hopelessly in conflict? Until fairly recently little effort was made, either by professionals or by parents, to change attitudes or behavior. Within the past decade or so, parents have become actively involved in social movements to bring about change. Recently too, new professional training curricula are being designed to promote awareness of the needs of children with disabilities and their families. Although professionals can never completely "walk in the shoes" of the families they serve, they can improve their "role-taking ability" through experiences that make them more aware of the life situations of families. Models that provide such experiences are the subject of this book.

Parent Activism

Consumerism in general has been growing in recent years. Various minority groups have also become more vocal in demanding their rights. As part of this larger social movement, parents of children with disabilities have become more active in asserting their demands for programs and services for their children. This new assertiveness has been aided by legislation such as the Education for All Handicapped Children Act (P.L. 94-142) and its amendments (P.L. 99-457)—now the Individuals with Disabilities Education Act (IDEA).

So far, most parental challenges have occurred within the realm of education. With the support of recent legislation, parents are confronting school administrators with demands for appropriate educational programs for their children. Challenges in the medical realm have not been as common. Many parents are still intimidated by medical authority and are reluctant to confront physicians directly with their concerns. Consumerism in the health care field has been increasing, however, and parents will be more likely to challenge the medical profession directly as support for such challenges grows.

A number of studies have indicated that the professional dominance of physicians may have declined somewhat in recent years. Gallup and Harris polls (reported in Betz & O'Connell, 1983) show that the public's confidence in and respect for physicians have declined since 1950. In 1966, some 72 percent of the public expressed confidence in doctors, but only 43 percent expressed such confidence in 1975. Haug and Lavin wrote that, "in the dialectic of power relations, the increasing monopolization of medical knowledge and medical practice could only call forth a countervailing force in the form of patient consumerism" (1983, p. 16). Consumerism is fostered further by interaction in self-help groups and by stories about successful advocacy efforts printed in the general media and specialized publications, such as *Exceptional Parent* magazine. (For a further discussion of parent activism, see Darling, 1988.)

Changing Professional Attitudes

In a number of fields, professionals have been moving away from a strict clinical focus and toward a "social system perspective" (Mercer, 1965). In the clinical perspective, the "official" (professional) definition of a family's situation is assumed to be the correct one. The social system perspective, on the other hand, "attempts to see the definition of an individual's behavior as a function of the values of the social system within which he is being evaluated." Clinical modes of treatment focus on changing the child (through medical or surgical procedures, education, or therapy) or the family (through counseling, "parent training," or other means). Professionals with a social system perspective are more likely to accept a family's views or preferences and to work toward creating services to improve the family's situation.

This shift in perspectives is especially evident in the early intervention field, where teachers and therapists have been moving toward a "family-centered" service system. As the author recently noted elsewhere (Darling & Darling, 1992), a number of factors have contributed to this shift, including the close working relationships that have developed between early interventionists and families, parent activism, and literature by parents and professionals. The field's new focus on families' resources, priorities, and concerns received legal sanction with the passage of Part H of Public Law (P.L.) 99-457 in 1986. The law has also been the impetus for increasingly strong efforts to include families in the planning and implementation of early intervention services at the federal, state, and local levels.

In the medical realm, a similar shift in perspectives has been evolving as part of the family-centered care movement. This movement recognizes that "families are the primary caregivers and advocates for their children" and encourages parent–professional collaboration rather than professional dominance (Hostler, 1991). "Within this philosophy is the idea that families should be supported in their natural care-giving and decision-making roles by building on their unique strengths as people and families" (Brewer, McPherson, Magrab & Hutchins, 1989). Family-centered care has been incorporated into the 1989 amendments to Title V of the Social Security Act.

The U.S. Bureau of Maternal and Child Health has been providing funding for various initiatives, including the Center for Family-Centered Care at the Association for the Care of Children's Health and various "Special Projects of Regional and National Significance," including physician training projects in several states. The Healthy Tomorrows Partnership between the Maternal and Child Health Bureau and the American Academy of Pediatrics requires that all funded projects be "community-based, family-centered, comprehensive and culturally relevant." In a recent article, Ireys and Nelson (1992) have suggested that pediatric training programs at all levels will need to incorporate the principles of community-based, family-centered care into their curricula.

OVERVIEW OF THE BOOK

The chapters are divided into three parts: (1) The Family's Perspective; (2) Models of Health Provider Education; and (3) Directions in Medical Education and Family-centered Care: Prospects for the 1990s and Beyond. Following these parts is a resource list of materials that are available for use in physician training programs.

The first part includes three chapters. Chapter 2, "Collaboration Defined Mathematically," is an edited transcript of Florene Poyadue's keynote address at the Pittsburgh conference that led to this book. In this chapter, Poyadue describes the necessary components of good relationships between parents and professionals. In Chapter 3, Sharon Spano, the parent of a child with special health needs, writes about her experience and offers some suggestions for professionals. In Chapter 4, Stanley Klein, using a psychologistic perspective, suggests strategies that promote better parent–professional communication, especially in the diagnostic situation.

The second part of the book is divided into two subparts. The first subpart includes three chapters on preservice models of health provider education. Chapter 5, written by Judy Lewis and Robert Greenstein, describes a course for first-year medical students at the University of Connecticut, in which the students spend time with families of children with disabilities. The authors include material from students and families illustrating the value of this experience so early in the students' medical careers. In Chapter 6, Nancy DiVenere describes the Medical Education Project of Parent to Parent of Vermont, in which parents are used as "community faculty" for medical students. In Chapter 7, Carl Cooley describes a number of medical residency programs that have incorporated into their curricula experiences with families in community-based settings.

The other subpart in Part II is on continuing education models and contains three chapters, all of which present models for training practicing physicians in the community. In Chapter 8, Margo Peter and Calvin Sia describe Hawaii's Medical Home Project, which has been replicated in a number of other states. The Hawaii model provides in-depth training to community physicians about the "medical home" concept and family-centered care. In Chapter 9, I describe a video-based model designed to reach large numbers of community physicians in a minimum amount of time. This model, which is based on research about physicians' reluctance to diagnose developmental disabilities, makes physicians aware of a "no-diagnosis" option they can use in referral to early intervention programs. Chapter 10, by Francine Gallagher and Corinne Garland, describes a study conducted in Virginia to determine physicians' perceived training needs. The authors describe a curriculum based on this assessment.

The third and final part of the book consists of two chapters. In Chapter 11, Alfred Healy discusses basic principles of health care for children with disabilities, as well as goals the health care system will need to adopt in order to implement these principles in the years ahead. Healy's chapter is a transcription of his general session address at the Pittsburgh conference. In Chapter 12, Margo Peter and I review all the previous chapters to answer the question "Where have we come from?" and, based on this review, to suggest future directions for work in this field.

We are at an exciting time in the history of health care for children in general and children with special needs in particular. As I write this, the federal government is moving toward universal immunization of children and universal health care. Support for family-centered care is greater than at any time in the past. Within this context, physicians have the potential to provide a level of care that truly meets the needs of all children and their families. Training health care providers to fulfill that potential is one of our greatest challenges in the years ahead.

NOTE

1. The following section is based largely on "Parent–Professional Interaction: The Roots of Misunderstanding," previously published by the author (Darling, 1991).

REFERENCES

Betz, M., & O'Connell, L. (1983). Changing doctor–patient relationships and the rise in concern for accountability. *Social Problems* 31:84–95.

Blackard, M. K., & Barsch, E. T. (1984). Parents' and professionals' perceptions of the handicapped child's impact on the family. *TASH Journal* 7:62–70.

Brewer, E. J., Jr., McPherson, M., Magrab, P. R., & Hutchins, V. L. (1989). Family-centered, community-based, coordinated care for children with special health care needs. *Pediatrics* 83:1055–1060.

Claflin, C. J., & Meisels, S. J. (1993). Assessment of the impact of very low birth weight infants on families. In N. J. Anastasiow & S. Harel, eds., *At-risk infants: Interventions, families and research*. Baltimore: Paul H. Brookes, pp. 57–79.

Darling, R. B. (1979). *Families against society: A study of reactions to children with birth defects*. Beverly Hills, CA: Sage.

Darling, R. B. (1988). Parental entrepreneurship: A consumerist response to professional dominance. *Journal of Social Issues* 44:141–158.

Darling, R. B. (1991). Parent–professional interaction: The roots of misunderstanding. In M. Seligman, ed., *The family with a handicapped child*, 2nd ed. Needham Heights, MA: Allyn & Bacon, pp. 119–149.

Darling, R. B., & Darling, J. (1982). *Children who are different: Meeting the challenges of birth defects in society*. St. Louis: C. V. Mosby.

Darling, R. B., & Darling, J. (1992). Early intervention: A field moving toward a sociological perspective. *Sociological Studies of Child Development* 5:9–22.

Francis, V., Korsch, B. M., & Morris, M. J. (1968). Gaps in doctor–patient communication: Patients' response to medical advice. *New England Journal of Medicine* 280:535–540.

Freidson, E. (1961). *Patients' views of medical practice*. New York: Russell Sage.

Freidson, E. (1970). *Professional dominance*. Chicago: Aldine.

Haug, M. R., & Lavin, B. (1983). *Consumerism in medicine: Challenging physician authority*. Beverly Hills, CA: Sage.

Hickson, G. B., Altemeier, W. A., & O'Connor, S. (1983). Concerns of mothers seeking care in private pediatric offices: Opportunities for expanding services. *Pediatrics* 72:619–624.

Hostler, S. L. (1991). Family-centered care. *Pediatric Clinics of North America* 38:1545–1560.

Ireys, H. T., & Nelson, R. P. (1992). New federal policy for children with special health care needs: Implications for pediatricians. *Pediatrics* 90:321–327.

Mercer, J. R. (1965). Social system perspective and clinical perspective: Frames of reference for understanding career patterns of persons labeled as mentally retarded. *Social Problems* 13:18–34.

Parsons, T. (1951). *The social system*. New York: Free Press.

Richardson, S. A. (1972). People with cerebral palsy talk for themselves. *Developmental Medicine and Child Neurology* 14:524–535.

Seligman, M., & Darling, R. B. (1989). *Ordinary families, special children: A systems approach to childhood disability*. New York: Guilford.

Sloper, P., & Turner, S. (1991). Parental and professional views of the needs of families with a child with severe physical disability. *Counselling Psychology Quarterly* 4:323–330.

Spina Bifida Association of America. (1982). Mother expresses serious concerns about catheterization program. *Spina Bifida Insights*, p. 9.

Stacey, M. (1980). Charisma, power, and altruism: A discussion of research in a developmental centre. *Sociology of Health and Illness* 2:64–90.

Stimson, G., & Webb, B. (1975). *Going to see the doctor: The consultation process in general practice*. London: Routledge & Kegan Paul.

Strong, P. M. (1979). *The ceremonial order of the clinic: Parents, doctors, and medical bureaucracies.* London: Routledge & Kegan Paul.

Wolraich, M. L. (1980). Pediatric practitioners' knowledge of developmental disabilities. *Journal of Developmental and Behavioral Pediatrics* 1:133–136.

Part I

The Family's Perspective

2

Collaboration Defined Mathematically

Florene Stewart Poyadue

This chapter is a transcription of Ms. Poyadue's keynote address given at the conference, "Creating Family–Professional Partnerships: Educating Physicians and Other Health Professionals to Care for Children with Chronic and Disabling Conditions," Pittsburgh, Pennsylvania, May 21–22, 1992.

I thank you for this opportunity to come and share at this unique conference. You have afforded me the opportunity to talk about one of my favorite subjects, which is parent–professional collaboration.

The reason parent–professional collaboration is so high on my list is that, as I am sure you realize, the primary reason for parent–professional collaboration is that it benefits the child. Caring for children is what parent–professional collaboration is really all about. At Parents Helping Parents, a parent-directed family resource center in San Jose, we feel that the key to bridging the gap between parents and professionals involves communication, education, and utilization of parents and professionals.

Because I'm a nurse, the first training I wanted to do when we first started, sixteen years ago, was with health care professionals. To that end I wrote a little book called *Better Ways: Training Physicians in Breaking Diagnostic News*. [See the Resource List at the end of this book.] It's really great to see that the rest of the world is catching up with Parents Helping Parents, as we implement this type of training. The first thing that I emphasized with physicians was that the main thing parents were interested in was that professionals listen to them. This doesn't even cost money. It requires only change in thought processes and attitudes. The other thing that I emphasized with physicians was the real importance of parent-to-parent contact. Families need to be connected to other families—not just so that they can get support, but so that they have access to the vast amount of information that experienced parents have to share with new parents. I found out later that there are three elements to recovery for people who have been traumatized. One element is to be allowed to help someone else who has been through a similar situation. The other two elements are to be dealt with in an empathetic manner and to have someone validate the difficulty of your experience. I find that parents are the ones who can do this best. The early training I did went over very well with physicians. They responded with everything from tears, to "nobody ever told me that there were better ways of breaking news to people," to real commitment to referring families to the family resource center and to collaborating with families.

Collaboration implies the mutual utilization of each other's knowledge, talents, experience, and expertise toward a common goal. Of course, in our case, the focus of commonality is the child with special needs. Today we want to take a look at what collaboration is, what the barriers and benefits are, how it changes roles, and why anyone would want to collaborate in the first place.

Do you feel like you are hearing the word *collaboration* an awful lot these days? Sometimes I feel that, if I hear it one more time, I'm just going to throw it out the window. We're saturated with hearing the word *collaboration.* We need to know that, most often, when we're hearing something an awful lot it's because it's not happening. I used to say to people, "When was the last time you heard me complaining about sitting at the back of the bus?" You don't have to hear that anymore because I'm no longer sitting there. Once we really have parent–professional collaboration, we won't have to talk about it so much; it will be happening.

Let's take a couple of quick looks at examples of what people thought was collaboration, but perhaps was not. My child's teacher listened intently as I talked to her about my son at our IEP (Individual Education Plan) team meeting, and I explained and shared information about him and what I felt his goals should be and our objectives on how we would get there. Then she proceeded to outline his IEP. She did not include or utilize my shared information. What we had was not a failure to communicate; we were communicating, but we were not collaborating. Another example of what it isn't, is the health care professional who tells parents how their child is doing, and explains the discharge plan that they (the professionals) have devised. Again, they have communicated, but not collaborated. In some instances we go a step further; we not only communicate with someone, but we get them to cooperate with us. I remember the days with one teacher when first she would communicate and tell us what was going on. Then there came a point in time when she would send some papers home, and I would have to cooperate by doing some of the things that were on the little purple sheets. Then we got to a point where we needed to collaborate. Let me give a little example. My son came home with a little purple sheet and it said, "Please have Dean go over rhyming, because he does not understand rhyming. [My son, Dean, just happens to have Down syndrome.] Have him draw the lines from cat to hat and mouse to house, etc." So we had him draw some lines and then we started to play some games in the kitchen while I was cooking. I said, "Oh, your sister Jill forgot to take her pill," and Dean played along, and began rhyming with me. I thought, "Gosh, I believe he does understand rhyming." So at that point we had communicated and I was cooperating, but I thought, "Now it's time to collaborate." So I went in and I said, "You know, I know he has shown you that he does not know rhyming. But at home he's showing me that he does." Notice that I went in accepting the fact that he was presenting to her the picture that she saw, hoping that she would also accept the picture that he was presenting to me. So, on a positive note of communication, I said, "But I think we need to take a look at how we have decided and defined that this is the problem." When you collaborate, you need to help define the problem together, as well as solve the problem. When we examined it together, we realized that Dean thought that every rodent was a rat, just because we see big rats around our house. He didn't know that other people have little ones, and that a little one might be called a "mouse." Therefore he would never draw a line from a rat to a house. He also wears eyeglasses. We found that, if he got the last mimeograph sheet, sometimes he couldn't see. So we knew then that he did not know that some animals have two or three different names, and he didn't know the names of some animals. He also needed bigger pictures and he needed to get really clear pictures. Now we were defining new problems. He knew rhyming, but he had these other problems. She said, "Well, if he doesn't know the animals, he can come up and ask me and I will tell him." Would Dean come up? No. Now we have another problem: assertiveness training for this child. Isn't this getting to be different when we're collaborating? I can assure you that the same thing happens in the health care field, in the educational field, in the social field. We came up with new goals, new objectives, ways of working with him, and so it was a different picture. It was really exciting. We were collaborating.

We have come a long way in our relationships. Parents and professionals are definitely communicating and cooperating. But family-centered, community-based, culturally competent coordinated care—as Dr. C. Everett Koop taught us—demands that we go further. This means increasing interaction between parents and professionals for better care of the child and optimum functioning and survival of the entire family. This includes considering the welfare of the siblings and of mom and dad as a couple. Families must be invited, encouraged, and, if necessary, taught in areas of planning, problem definition and resolution, and implementation of care and services. How can we start this wonderful process?

Most parents want to collaborate, I believe. However, many professionals (if they dare to risk honesty) find that they are at least skeptical about this thing called "collaboration." I can think of several ways to engender the professionals' interest in collaboration. A couple of them are pretty drastic. One would be to just hit them over the head, but I don't think we want to do that. Another would be to have every professional give birth to a child with special needs. Then they would be in the category called "parents," which would also put them in the category of wanting to collaborate. I think both of those are a little bit drastic. What we *can* do is to interest professionals in a conscious choice for change. And we could also introduce them to some of the great benefits and the good by-products of collaboration. These include less frustration in their relationships with parents, more knowledge and resources at their fingertips (you'll find that parents have a lot of information that can be beneficial), better interagency networking; trust is up. When this happens, money is saved. Parents are often the cheapest experts on the market; they often work free. Just ask.

The main barriers to the wonderful process lie mired in our myths about people and each other. These myths are fed by fears, and inflamed by fragile egos of insecure individuals. Many myths are inherent in the titles or labels that we apply to people. These labels seem to stick like superglue. Once you're labeled a professional or a parent, whatever else it is you were or you could do is totally forgotten.

This even happens when we confer the label *parent*. Sometimes it seems that the moment a woman goes into labor a strange transformation occurs. She is transferred to the labor room where she delivers the child; out comes the child, out comes the placenta, and then out comes her brain. Now you have what you call a "parent," which is an emotional, brainless being. A woman has been transformed into a mom. The other myth is that as you become a professional, you complete school, get your sheepskin, and you gain a big salary and you lose your heart. (Of course, nobody's seen your check recently, so, you know, they don't know about the big-salary part.)

Now what you have is a rich heartless perfectionist called a "professional." Born out of these myths are statements like, "Parents won't be able to understand," and, "Professionals don't really care." Both are true some of the time, and both are false most of the time. What we want to be sure of is that we are not guilty of judging the many by the few on either side.

Fear is also a great barrier to parent–professional collaboration. Fear tangles the tongues of people—parents and professionals. Collaboration requires open, honest communication. Some parents don't communicate openly and honestly for fear that they might anger a professional, who will then be left in charge of their child. Though this may be an unfounded fear, parents have it and professionals must realize it. Parents may worry that you will retaliate using their child if they upset your apple cart. Some professionals fear the wrath of their colleagues and their superiors. I have had my professional friends suggest that a child's needs' assessment should somehow be connected to what an agency's budget can afford in the way of services. I have suggested to them that we have a neutral assessment team who will have nothing to do with the services that the child gets, so that they look at him and consider his needs without worrying about what the budget is.

Both professionals and parents are made dysfunctional by fragile egos and pride that causes them to fight to maintain an appearance of perfection. Ah, the tyranny of perfection. When I did training with physicians fourteen years ago, I had them practice saying "I don't know." I start my training of physicians with a little quiz. I give them twenty quick questions about services in town, families' needs, and where they would find various things for their patients and their families. Then I tell them just to put it away. Well, many of them immediately say, "We want to know these answers." As I give those answers, a dialogue between the two of us begins. Then we get to the point of them practicing saying "I don't know." Many physicians have said to me that they feel, if they say "I don't know," then people won't respect them and that they will lose credibility. I hear just the opposite from parents. They say they love it if a professional admits that they're human and that they don't know.

As professionals, it's hard to say "I don't know." We all want to be perfect. We all want to know. So we even have to practice it sometimes. Some people never get started on what they need to do in life, because their plan must be perfect, and they keep massaging the plan, and nothing else gets done but the massaging of the plan. So the tyranny of perfection halts us in our tracks and immobilizes us. Sheldon Kopp writes, "When you see Buddha on the road, kill him." The most pervasive neurosis of our time is the need to be special, the goal of being perfect, the idea that anything less than perfect is failure. Fear can rule our lives, because we're probably not going to be perfect. We are afraid to collaborate because we're afraid to make a change. So fear has a lot to do with our failure to collaborate.

But collaboration does not require perfection. We don't have to be perfect to collaborate. Do keep in mind that people who are competent and secure and self-assured have the qualities that can afford them the luxury of sharing their power and letting go of control. Change in a system must start with individuals making a change in themselves. Therefore, a large part of the answer to the problems of parents and professionals working together lies within each person—in eliminating his or her own insecurities, honing their own skills, raiding their self-assuredness, and increasing their self-esteem to such a level that others will say of us, in this day and time, that the only thing that exceeds our competence, our compassion, and our caring is our ability to collaborate.

So we are faced with change, and with change comes the dis-ease of change. Let's spend a little time looking at normalizing that dis-ease of change. The dis-ease of change comes from not knowing ourselves and not knowing our own values, and not knowing our own choices. Change—listen to this because this is important and I think this is what happens to a lot of us, because we are forced by laws and by mandates to collaborate, and so we try to make a change that is not based on our own inner needs, or our own goals, and it's false, and it's faulty, and it's painful. Therefore, it produces anxious, confused, and disillusioned individuals. When you make a change, you should expect to go through the loss/grief process. Why is that? Because you are grieving the loss of the familiar. The moment someone starts to talk to you about a change, the first thing that usually happens is that you will deny that it is even needed. There's a tendency to say, "Why, we're doing what we do and it's been fine so far. Why do we need change?" And just watch this the next time, whether it's in your office or with your family or whatever, that you start talking about a change; people will start going into this grief/loss process. And then they will get angry because they think you are stepping on their toes and entering their territory and you're saying that what they did before was not right. They will start bargaining with you: "Well, if you're going to make this change, please make it quick or make it simple," or whatever. And they will get depressed because it looks like you're going to go ahead and make this change anyway, and in five years they will accept the change, and ten years from now they will really appreciate the fact that you made the change. So when you hear someone start to go into denial and anger when you start talking about a change, be happy. You know that the process has begun, and that they have to go through that.

How can we normalize this dis-ease of change? And why do I dwell on change in the first place? Because if we're going to collaborate, we're going to have to switch to this new collaborative mode, where the professional goes from being the sage on stage to being the guide at the side, and that's a real change. And becoming collaborative means being a systems change agent. So, as we look at normalizing the dis-ease of change, a strange way of putting it might be to have people understand that the normal side effects of change include such things as discomfort, fear, disorientation, feelings of insecurity and confusion. It is okay, as it were, to feel ill at ease with questions about how you will negotiate, survive, and endure this dis-ease of behavioral changes. Kind of like a pregnant woman who is about to give birth, and she knows—at least she should know—that there's going to be some pain involved. I always have to broaden the smile on my face when I think of how men talk about labor pains and they speak of the "discomfort" that their wife had, as they understate what the pain was. Only a man would call labor pains "discomfort." I talk about it as a flash flood of pain, and from those first contractions she knows that this dis-ease is a part of the adventure and experience. She is committed to getting a job done. A problem arises, though—sometimes—in being so committed to an old behavior that we feel disloyal trying a new one. It would be like this expectant mother getting so hooked on being pregnant that she would refuse to submit to labor and delivery. We don't want to be that way about our old rules and regulations. We must submit to the pains of change.

Some think that the new behavior—if it is good, then the old one must have been rotten and therefore *they* must have been rotten, and they start to equate the behavior with themselves. Not having developed a life strategy that gives flexibility, a single-minded devotion to past incantations from old authority figures and methods of operating gets in our way. Not knowing what one really wants, questioning priorities, being frightened by our lifelong assumptions, we choose to make hurdles in our environment rather than having a smooth running course.

Do we believe in collaboration? To improve our chances for changing, we can realize that, number one, making a change with an inadequate amount of information is uncomfortable. Undeveloped planning skills make it uncomfortable, and labeling changes as a threat instead of an opportunity makes it uncomfortable. Mendosa and Stevens at the University of San Diego talked a lot and wrote a lot about collaboration.

They said the main skills and attitudes necessary to make collaboration work are: mutual respect, a desire to work together, honest communication, that we acknowledge and consider the point of view of others, and that we use creative problem-solving approaches.

I did some soul-searching with myself, and that's always nice—I get a chance to talk to someone who's intelligent for a change. Actually, I did most of the soul-searching with my twenty-one-year-old son who just happened to be awake with me one night at midnight. And I was thinking about this thing, collaboration. And I thought that most of the time we hear about *what* it is, which is kind of what we've gone through this morning, and we also get some skills on *how* to go about it; and then it dawned on us that maybe *why* is the thing that is keeping people from doing the collaboration. *Why* would you want to collaborate in the first place? And so we looked at those five main skills that Jeanne Mendosa and Trudy Stevens had come up with, and we looked at number one. It says *mutual respect*, that we need to give each other mutual respect. Why would we want to give someone mutual respect? We might do it if we view them as competent in an area in which we would like to have some information, or an area that we might be interested in. So we might all start to be more collaboratively attractive ourselves by being more competent. I like that term, "collaboratively attractive." You make yourself collaboratively attractive so others will be attracted to you. Difference is another reason you might respect another person's opinion. Even though you don't agree with it, the difference you just might find refreshing. You don't have to agree with everything that is different. Also, if you learn to value and appreciate difference, then you might be willing to respect another person's ideas. We also realize that selfish or self-centered people have a hard time respecting others. Why? Because all praise needs to come to them, the people who are self-centered. Therefore, it is difficult to collaborate if the person you're collaborating with is going to start to get some of the praise. How much do you need all of the praise? How much can you share the spotlight?

So, what do we need to do to become more collaboratively attractive? Become less selfish. Be willing to share the praise. I would like to see us start saturating each other with care and praise. That's something that we can easily do. We can start by giving others some praise so that they will have enough to give away.

When we looked at the *desire to work together*, we thought, "What the heck can make us want to work together?" We can learn to get acquainted with other facts that we do not have, if we work together and if we realize that others often act as a catalyst for our own development for our highest potential. The more I collaborate with other people, the more I have the opportunity for them to boost my excellence. So this again—if you are a bit selfish, here is a selfish reason to collaborate. If you want someone to collaborate with you, concentrate on helping that person to blossom into their fullest bloom, and hopefully someone else will do the same for you. In the same vein, realize that you are closing off an avenue for your own potential development when you close off collaboration. People often talk about two heads are better than one, but I do like to add—and I think people find this rather refreshing—that sometimes two heads are not better than one. How many of you have thought that, at times? There are times when you could come up with a better solution on your own, and in half the time, than if you got together with four other people. I promise you that. Now, why then would you want to get together with these four other people? One of the reasons is, if these four other people have to be involved in the implementation of that solution. It is better to have a solution that is 75 percent correct and people buying in 100 percent, than to have a 100-percent-correct solution and them sabotaging it or buying in at only 50 percent. This is why you go toward consensus and collaboration—not always because they will come up with a better solution as a group. You can practice that, if you would like, by giving five people a riddle to solve, and put five of them in five different rooms; and then put five people together in one room, and give them the riddle to solve. And probably the five people in one room will solve the riddle faster. So you can oftentimes save some time by a collaborative effort.

They also ask us to risk *honesty.* Why would you want to risk honesty in your communications with anyone, especially with a stranger? Sometimes, for the family, this is the first time they're coming to the physician; or for the nurse or the teacher it's the first time that they're seeing this family—and they're going to ask you to risk honesty? Do you know at what level of communication risking honesty is? It's about the sixth level of communication. Therefore we have to work our way back and up again in order to get to risking honesty. When we look at it, we see that honest communication is the sixth level—what is the fifth level? We have to reach the fifth level before we can reach the sixth level, and the fifth level is creating trust. You've got to trust people before you can risk honesty. Now, how did you get to trust? You have to share information, and share thoughts, and share feelings; and sharing is the fourth level. Once you do the fourth level, you get the trust which will lead to the sixth. So we're asking you to start at six—I'm telling you you've got to back up. What about the third step before you can start sharing? You have to meet; you have to spend some time together. And what about the second level—how are you going to get together and spend time together? You have to plan it. Someone has to plan it, like someone had to plan this conference. So now we spend some time together, we share some information, we will build some trust, and we will start being honest with each other. Why would you want to bring people together in the first place? Why did they bring us together here? Because you have a common focus, a common reason. So this is what collaboration is all about. We have to realize that one of the reasons that people don't do this step is that we're asking them to start out on the sixth level of communication. So back up and work your way up and you will be able to answer that "why."

Why would you want to *consider other people's points of view* when you're always totally right in the first place? And why do you need to listen to these other people? Even though you're all right, there is more rightness to know about. I'd like for you to do a little game with me once more. I'd like for you to build a perception scope. You just build that out of your fist. You just make a fist like this and you look through it and up here toward the podium, and you see one beautiful black lady, right? That's all you see, and that is correct, and that is all good knowledge. That is your perception. But it is limited. Now if you open your perception scope, open it up, you also see a beautiful white lady that's sitting up here; so there is more information. This came home to me when I was at a meeting trying to plan for children's care. There was a nurse from a tertiary hospital setting coming up with wonderful, wonderful ideas. We only had ninety minutes to come up with some beginnings of a plan. She had to stop to take a breath for a minute; and when she did, someone else got a chance to interject something else; and it hit her like a bolt of lightning. She leaned over and said, "Oh, my gosh, I've been hogging the conversation." She said that was wonderful information. I said, "Yes, but everything you were saying was wonderful information and everything you were saying was correct. What you just realized is that there are other segments. There's the home, and there's the clinics, and there's the school nurse, and there's the public health nurse." So, we get so focused in on our perception. And it is true: The information we have is correct. But there is more correct information out there. So let's learn to broaden our perception scopes.

Using *creative problem solving*, as I mentioned, can save us time and lead to better solutions. And we do want to learn to negotiate if we're going to collaborate, because negotiation leads to a win/win situation. People do need to tell you that collaboration takes time, and that you do need to have a healthy ego, because there will be people who will steal your ideas and take credit for it. That's all right if you can grow that kind of a healthy ego.

But I would like to conclude with a couple of things. One is what I call the "chemistry of collaboration," and another little bit about the math. I write poetry in my spare time, so I wouldn't want you to get away without a little poetry, because there's more to life than news, weather, and sports. We look at the chemistry of collaboration. I see it as being a catalyst for change, for speeding and improving interactions between the magic ingredients—the ingredients are parents and professionals—to produce a new element, which is wonderful care for children. And when I speak mathematically of collaboration, I am talking about adding to each other's base of knowledge, subtracting our major differences, dividing the praise among you, and multiplying the benefits for our children. I think that we can get all of that done if we will take my "View in Miniature," which is a little poem that I wrote to keep my head in the right place.

View in Miniature

My eye beholds this earth
Like a microscope in reverse.
Though to most men we giants be,
This earth and the things herein
Are like tiny vagaries to me.
It can be frightening, though—
This view in miniature—
For, if a mountain range
An anthill seems,
And a saucer can't be filled by the sea,
How insignificant me.

3

The Miracle of Michael

Sharon L. Spano

Loss of the Dream Child

So you're going to have a baby!!! The news spreads. The father-to-be is beside himself with joy. Family and friends are ecstatic. This is the dream child you have been waiting for since you yourself were a little girl playing with dolls. At long last, you will become the perfect mom married to the ideal man. Together you will attain the American dream of a career, home, and two-point-five children. Preparations begin for this first dream child: Lamaze classes, wallpaper, baby clothes, wooden cradle. So much to do. You eat right, get plenty of rest, exercise, and wait. While you wait, you fantasize about who this dream child will be. Tennis star, astronaut, literary genius. You read volumes of books on childcare and parenting: how to bathe a newborn; the pros and cons of breast feeding; how to raise a more intelligent preschooler. A colicky baby is your worst fear. You take calligraphy classes to ensure that the baby announcements are a masterpiece. The pages in the book of names wear thin as you diligently search for a name worthy of the dream child. You wait. You dream. You wait some more. Only five more days until the due date—then you and your husband can resume a perfect life with the dream child. Everything is ready. You are prepared to receive this celebration of life!!!

Or are you? Wait. Is it possible you forgot to prepare for one very important thing? Is it possible you have made a terrible mistake in preparing for the ideal of a "perfect" child? The baby is born. "Something is not quite right," they say. Imperfect? How is this possible? We didn't prepare for imperfection! From the depths of your soul you silently scream, "No!" Your husband's eyes are dead. The world stops. The dream is shattered.

And so it is for hundreds of families each and every day as they suddenly meet the hard reality of what it will mean to face the challenge of rearing a child with special needs. The day my son Michael was born, the world did indeed seem to come to a screeching halt. I did not know at that moment that Michael would prove to be the most wonderful experience of my life. There was little hope that could be offered to my husband and me once we were informed that Michael would not live beyond the age of two. Numb with grief, we took our baby home and desperately tried to make sense of it all. Suddenly all the preparations that had been made seemed superfluous, and we were thrown into a complex medical system that was overwhelming and seemed to have little regard for what we were experiencing as parents. We began the task of trying to determine how best to meet the challenges ahead. We struggled to balance our unconditional love for our son with the horrific fear of losing him to some little-understood illness.

FAMILY-CENTERED CARE: A BETTER WAY OF WORKING WITH FAMILIES

Today, thanks to a paradigm shift in the way health care professionals and other service providers are addressing the unique strengths and needs of the family, our society finally acknowledges that there is no possible way for a family to prepare for, nor is there a "right way" for a family to meet, the diverse challenges of rearing a child with special needs. The philosophical understanding of "family-centered care" recognizes that there is no such thing as the ideal American family and that we cannot expect any family to conform to an ideal approach to child rearing. Rather, family-centered care recognizes the diverse nature of the family in our culture and further emphasizes that each and every family will nurture and respond to their child's needs in a variety of ways. Further, the family is valued as the constant in the child's life and respected for their expertise in addressing the unique needs of the child. There is no room for judgment within the philosophical framework of family-centered care since the loss of a dream child is a very personal experience for each family member.

Pain does not discriminate and pose the foolish questions, "Are you a single mom or a working father? Are you a man of wealth or a grandmother on state assistance? Are you a teen parent or a middle-aged father of two? Are you educated or illiterate? Are you black, white, yellow, or brown?" Pain knows no boundaries. Each family member must be afforded the opportunity to experience the loss of the dream child in his or her own way without judgment from the outside world. Consequently, the philosophical framework of family-centered care requires that providers value and respect the essential differences within the family unit and acknowledge that the family members' approaches to meeting the needs of the child will vary depending on where they are within this process.

Accordingly, the underlying premise of family-centered care is that *collaboration* between the family and the health care provider is vital to the health and well-being of the child. Providers are thereby encouraged to explore new ways of working with the family to facilitate a partnership that acknowledges the family as an equal partner in meeting the unique health care needs of the child.

According to recent teachings in family-centered care (Edelman, Greenland & Mills, 1992, p. 18), a collaborative partnership between the health care provider and the family can best be achieved when skills are demonstrated and valued in the following areas:

1. Building mutual trust and respect;
2. Clarifying roles and expectations;
3. Communication with families; and
4. Solving problems and resolving conflicts.

What does this mean in terms of day-to-day interactions with families? When health care providers are faced with the question of whether or not they are family centered in their daily interactions with families, their answer quite often is an unequivocal yes. Obviously, the very nature of the discipline implies that health care providers have the innate ability to meet the needs of children and families within the philosophical framework of family-centered care. Unfortunately, however, if the same question were to be placed before a group of family members who have encountered the medical community with any degree of regularity, the answer is most certain to be an unequivocal no. Where then lies the discrepancy? Are health care providers unresponsive and insensitive to the needs of the family? Or are family members so overwrought with their own circumstances that they are unable to appreciate fully the compassionate hand being offered? There is no black-and-white answer to these questions, perhaps, except to acknowledge that both the health care provider and the family are doing the best they can, given what they know at any specific moment in time. The ultimate challenge, then, is for each to learn to value and appreciate the vital role that the other plays in meeting the health care needs of the child.

While health care providers are cognizant of the fact that the family's experience of the medical community is often colored by where the family is within the grieving process, it is important to realize that the family's interpretation of the event is *real* for the family at that point in time and must be appreciated as such. Consider for a moment the scenario of a young child waking in the middle of the night, terrified by a nightmare. In much the same way that one would innately value the importance of offering comfort—not ridicule—to a child who experiences the terror of the night, so too must the health care provider be cautioned against invalidating the family's perception of the experience simply because that perception differs from his or her own. Accordingly, the health care provider is encouraged to meet the greater challenge of treating the family with dignity and respect during the family's most stressful moments—those in which the health care provider sees the family in anger, denial, or frustration. It is simply too easy to turn off the light, slam the door, and tell them the nightmare isn't real. Much like the terrors that make the child cry out for help, the nightmarish complexities of the medical community are very real to the family and should not be treated lightly by the health care professional simply because he or she has become accustomed to the inner workings of the system. Often the best way to offer some ray of hope that dawn will come is for the health care provider simply to acknowledge, by his or her actions, that where the family finds itself in its experience is okay. The manner in which health care providers respond to the family during moments of crisis can be a critical factor in how the family responds to the ongoing challenges of rearing a child with special needs.

BUILDING A PARTNERSHIP WITH FAMILIES

Let us explore the four basic areas that can assist the health care provider in establishing a collaborative relationship with the family: (1) building mutual trust and respect; (2) clarifying roles and expectations; (3) communication with families; and (4) solving problems and resolving conflicts. I will offer my own personal experiences with the use of examples (and nonexamples) in an effort to give the health care provider some insight into at least one family scenario; and I ask that these examples be valued beyond the scope of one family, as a means of demonstrating the impact that health care providers have on *all* families when they are faced with the complexities of the medical community. Again, I reiterate that my memories are based on my experience of the circumstances at a particular point in time and, while they may not be reflective of how the events actually occurred, it is important to realize that the following recollections serve as representations of how specific events have become an indelible memory over the years.

Building Mutual Trust and Respect

Mutual trust and respect must be the foundation for a collaborative relationship between the health care provider and the family. I have often heard family members discuss how intimidated they are by the medical professionals who seem to buzz in and out of their lives. Conversely, providers share that they often only see a family on one or two occasions, and that time constraints do not always afford the opportunity for the establishment of a relationship with the family. It is important to remember that the philosophical framework of family-centered care encourages health care providers to go beyond time and the logistical challenges of the system in their commitment to provide every child and family with options and the opportunity for an enhanced quality of life. It takes only a moment in time to acknowledge the innate goodness of another human being and to create a compassionate and caring atmosphere of mutual respect. A family member who feels that someone is willing to make an effort to work creatively in partnership toward a solution is far more likely to work with the system in a cooperative manner. Even the most frustrated individual will respond to unconditional kindness and respect.

The following recommendations are adapted from the Project Copernicus series on *Building Parent/Professional Collaboration* (Edelman, Greenland & Mills, 1992) and will assist health care providers in establishing a relationship with the family that is built on mutual trust and respect:

- Actively listen to the concerns and priorities of the family.
- Be open and honest with the family in sharing information.
- Follow through on the care coordination plans.
- Do not speak to family members in a condescending manner.

- Do not assume that only the health care provider knows what is best for the child.
- Acknowledge the innate ability of the family to do what is best for their child.
- Offer support and encouragement to the family.

In the following shared experience of my son Michael's first days of life, I invite you to consider how a health care provider might have better established mutual trust and respect with my family, using the above recommendations as a guide.

> Michael is only a few days old, and my husband and I are so scared we can hardly look each other in the eye. At night we sleep back to back without touching. I think we are so afraid that if we make any contact at all with each other we will break. I am trying to be strong for him and not let him see how terrified I am. He is doing the same for me, but I can feel his fear. I spend most of the day at the hospital, but we don't seem to be getting much information about what is really wrong with the baby. My husband runs back and forth between the hospital and the office. It's hard to believe that only a few short days ago we were an exuberant young couple with the world at our feet. Today I feel as though we have each lived two lifetimes. Our son looks so small and frail in the intensive care unit. We feel so helpless. There is a sign in the unit that reads: "Forty-five days to bankruptcy." I'm not sure the purpose of this sign, but it has us frantically worried about what we will do if Michael is here for an extended period of time. My husband says we'll sell the house and everything we have, if necessary. Our entire lives seem to have been turned upside down in just a matter of days. It's all so very frightening. I overheard the nurses say that they might transfer Michael to Children's Hospital downtown, but no one has said why. Friends don't seem to know what to say to us. I sit in the nursery with the sunlight filtering through the eyelet curtains my best friend so lovingly made and I blankly stare at the angelic faces of the children on the carefully selected wallpaper, wondering what lies ahead. . . .
>
> They have moved him. It broke my heart to know he had ridden in a big ambulance without us to comfort him or to be at the other hospital when he arrived. We didn't know he had been moved until later that evening. When I walked into the unit, there was a group of doctors standing around him. I saw Michael lying on his stomach, and he tried to lift his head a little. I thought that was amazing for a newborn. There was a moment of hope. Then I heard the doctors say

he was pretty strong for a "cardiac baby." Cardiac baby! My cardiologist told me he had a slight heart murmur. Lots of people have heart murmurs—but cardiac baby! What do they mean? My husband and I feel so empty without him at home. How is it possible that you can miss someone who has never been in your life before now? . . .

He's coming home. Thank God. My cardiologist says that he has a possible coarctation of the aorta and might need surgery later on. This doctor was so good at explaining to us what that meant, and he even drew us a diagram. He has kind eyes and speaks to us with such compassion. I can tell by his eyes that he really wants to help Michael. He always returns my calls even if it's ten o'clock at night. I am amazed how long his days are and thankful that he makes the time for us. I am afraid to take a shower or let Michael out of my sight for one moment, for fear he will stop breathing or something much worse. No one gave me any special instructions on his care, so I tell myself that whatever I do will be the right thing. It's so hard to really enjoy him when I feel as if his life is in my hands. The sweet innocence of him in my arms gives me strength. . . .

I took the baby to the pediatrician today for the first time and cried all the way home. The doctor was so abrupt in his handling of Michael as he tossed him around like a rag doll. After having undergone so many tests at the hospital, Michael was shaking with fear. I stood there stupefied by the doctor's insensitivity. I guess he is simply accustomed to shrieking babies. I thought I had prepared myself to be a good mother, but I felt so incompetent as he abruptly stated that Michael has probably not gained any weight because I am breastfeeding instead of using a formula. I am horrified with the thought, and remember how I struggled to get to the hospital to nurse Michael while he was in the ICU. I was so upset when I left the pediatrician's office that I phoned my cardiologist, wailing like a fool. Who is this woman? I used to be so in control. This doctor is my light in the darkness. He calmly told me to get another pediatrician. He said Michael may not gain much weight because of his heart condition. He reassured me that we are doing a great job of caring for Michael and not to worry. As soon as Michael is old enough for solid food, I'm going to make all of his meals from scratch so hopefully he will be better nourished and grow faster. He's doing so well now and is such a happy baby that the traumatic first days of his life seem long ago. . . .

My neighbor's baby is a few days older than Michael and doing so much more. I have read everything on developmental milestones and know that Michael should be crawling by now. My doctors keep telling me that he will outgrow this delay and that because he was in the hospital he will be a little slower in doing some things. I work with him every day—reading, playing, talking to him. He is so alert. I wonder if I am doing everything that I should be doing. He's still not growing. I have started a journal for Michael, describing how exciting each day is with him in my life. We are a family now. I make him outfits for every important sporting event. He looks so cute in his World Series shirt, and my husband and I marvel at how indulgent he is of his corny parents. We are laughing more now and becoming less and less fearful. . . .

We are moving across the country. It's a dream-come-true opportunity for us. My cardiologist insists on doing a routine echocardiogram before we leave. The moving van is being loaded. A phone call. The doctor is not comfortable with the echo. He insists on doing another heart catheterization before we leave for Florida. No!!!!! I feel sick inside. What is happening. I thought this was a common heart condition that Michael would either outgrow or that would possibly require surgery later. Arrangements are made to stay with friends. Flights are canceled. The nightmare begins again. . . .

He's down the hall. When they took him from us, he cried so hard I thought my heart would break. It was very helpful for us to see the room where they will be doing the catheterization. At least we were able to go in there with him beforehand. Maybe he won't be so scared since he's already seen the room and all the equipment. We are pacing like caged lions. My doctor said to wait in Michael's room, and they will bring him back to us after the catheterization is complete. We wait. We pace. We wait some more. The nurse says the doctor wants to see us right away outside the recovery room! What is happening!!! He told us they would bring Michael here. Something has gone wrong. The elevator won't come. It seems like an hour. Did his heart stop on the table? Oh, God, I feel as if I can't breathe—the fear is choking me. My husband has aged before my eyes. I, too, feel soooo very tired.

My doctor solemnly enters the room. His eyes are black with sorrow. I look into them, trying to find some reassurance. There is none. Michael is fine, for now. It is not a coarctation of the aorta. It is something of greater magnitude. A heart biopsy must be done. I hear something about cardiomyopathy. His eyes tell me he is having trouble telling me what all this might mean. The room seems so small. I hear him talking, but he sounds so far away. Something about surgery won't help. Something about the muscle of the heart. Michael may live until the age of two. Die! Did he say "Die"? How did we get from corrective surgery to DIE? Two years old! An image flashes through my mind of my two-year-old son in a coffin. I feel my husband beside me, not moving. He seems to shrink in the chair. I dare not look at him, for fear he is only two inches high. I reach for his hand. There is no strength in his powerful arm. He is weakened with grief. The room is silent. My doctor's eyes say he too is helpless. I am terrified to look into those eyes, but I must know more. I find the courage to speak from somewhere unknown to me, asking question after question. When should we do the biopsy? Who will do it? What is the procedure? What will be Michael's quality of life? On and on, and somehow together we make the necessary decisions and arrangements. I trust these eyes. We will return from our new home in Florida to do what must be done.

I hold my precious son in my arms for the next nine hours, never moving. We rock, and I count the flowers on the wallpaper. There are eight rows down and thirty-seven across. Over and over I count. My husband paces. We do not eat. We do not sleep. We are both dead inside. Michael in my arms is the only thing that is keeping me sane. The nurses are abruptly buzzing in and out to check on him. It's as though my husband and I do not exist. They seem not to notice our agony. I know they must do their job, but I long for a moment to cry in private. Today the journal stops. There is no more laughter.

The above example is intended to illustrate some of the subtle ways in which the medical community unknowingly causes the family to experience unnecessary anxiety and pain. I offer the following suggestions:

- Allow time for the family to talk openly about the concerns and worries for the child, and give them choices on how to best meet those challenges.
- Answer questions from the family in a clear and concise manner, using appropriate language and admitting when you do not know the answer.
- Remember that the family is struggling to balance their day-to-day living with the complexities of the newly experienced medical community. Dignify their efforts by assuming that each family member is doing the best he or she can.
- Do not impose your life choices or judgments on the family.
- Refer the family to local support organizations and acknowledge the positive efforts of the family and the successes of the child.
- Offer the family options for early intervention supports and services.

Clarifying Roles and Expectations

It is important to remember that encountering the challenging environment of the medical community is often an overwhelming experience for the family. Some providers are fortunate in that they have been afforded educational opportunities that gradually acclimate them to the complexities of the medical world, whereas the family is often thrust into the system with little or no preparation. For a family that is facing the diagnosis of a child with special health care considerations, the overwhelming *number* of professionals on the medical team, in and of itself, is often frightening since the family often has little understanding of who or even why specific individuals are involved in the care of their child. Consequently, there is a feeling of isolation from the medical team—a feeling that exacerbates the family's stress and anxiety. In a collaborative relationship, the health care provider is encouraged to assist the family in understanding the role of each member of the medical team and in clarifying the family's expectations for all involved in the care and well-being of the child.

Let us again look to what recommendations might be useful for the health care provider in meeting the goal of clarifying roles and expectations for the family.

- Identify your role as health care provider and clarify how you fit in with the team of providers.
- Clarify for the family all important information about the health care team.
- Ask the family relevant questions that will determine their expectations for the child and their expectations of the medical team.
- Determine the role of each family member in the care of the child.
- Establish for the family a contact person in your office.
- Record and file all information about the child and family, determining what has already taken place, what will happen next, and which member of the team is responsible for each action.
- Restate the care coordination plan at the end of the meeting with the family.

Even a routine examination by a medical team can result in undue stress on the family. The following experience will illustrate how easy it is for health care providers to unknowingly rob the family of dignity when there is failure to clarify roles and expectations.

> There is so much confusion. Each doctor tells me something different. My cardiologist in Florida tells me Michael's heart is within normal range and there is little need to worry. When I express anxiety about

Michael's inability to walk at nineteen months, he does not seem concerned. I recall the frightening conversation coming from my doctors in Los Angeles and New York and desperately try to make sense of it all. My husband prefers the Florida doctor because he seems more optimistic about Michael's future; however, I can't forget the sorrowful eyes of the cardiologist in Los Angeles. I wish they would talk to each other. I have requested that all communication between doctors be carbon copied to me, in the hopes of deciphering what is being said. They seem to communicate fine in writing; however, when I question the discrepancies between them, each invalidates the opinion of the other. It seems everyone wants to do his own version of the same test. I have purchased some medical dictionaries so I can better understand the terminology and discuss Michael's condition with my doctors on a more realistic level. I'm starting to wonder if perhaps Michael doesn't need to see some other specialists—neurologist, maybe? I keep asking my cardiologist, and he finally responds, "It's your dime. If you want to see one, go ahead." I want to trust him, but at the same time I don't feel that he is taking Michael's condition seriously enough. There is this sick feeling inside me that no one really cares if he is growing, walking, or talking. There are parts of him in research laboratories in three cities, yet we get no closer to understanding. Can it be they will only help me if he becomes critically ill and begins to deteriorate? I refuse to simply wait for him to die. A panicked call to Los Angeles confirms my worst fear.

"Come home," says Dr. Sorrow. He cannot believe that my doctors in Florida have not referred me to a neurologist and that Michael has not been in physical or occupational therapy. I feel so guilty inside and there is a deep sense of emptiness. I asked. I pleaded. I trusted them to lead me in the right direction. "Come as soon as you can. A muscle biopsy must be done." Will this nightmare ever end? . . .

Who are all these people? We were told to be at Children's Hospital by 7:00 A.M. to see the neurologist. We arrived a few days earlier in hopes that Michael would adjust to the time change before the biopsy, but he seems as exhausted as we are anxious. Throughout the day we wait. The elevator door opens a thousand times and each time my husband jumps up in anticipation of the doctor. He is not used to waiting. All day, people are in and out of the room, asking questions. At first I eagerly answer, hoping they are involved in Michael's care and will in turn share information; however, as the day wears on, it becomes clear to me that each is only passing through. I answer the same questions over and over again, hoping that what I am able to share might in some way help my little boy. The "busy people" shake their heads, scratch their chins, examine his little body over and over again, nodding to one another in intelligent agreement that he is indeed "interesting." Each time the busy people enter the room I see the terror in Michael's eyes, and I try to calm him by not letting him see the same fear in mine. Personal questions are repeatedly asked about our lives. My pregnancy and delivery are no longer the sacred experience they once were. As I hear myself recount what was once a joyous moment, I feel that memory fade and become forever tarnished by the deeper loss of the dream child. We are naked before the busy people; yet, when we ask questions in return, we are simply told they are "cautiously optimistic." They come and they go, leaving behind a hopeless sense that we are just one family among many.

As we anxiously await the elusive neurologist—still uncertain of why we are seeing him—I wonder if I am to become like the shadows of women I have met pacing the hospital corridors. They are aged with worry and they talk of returning year after year to nurture their children in illness. There is no evidence in this place of the dignity of the glorious experience of motherhood, and I am beginning to realize that these halls filled with busy people will soon rob me of my own joy if I am not careful. I hold Michael close to me and console myself with the sweetness of his dark curly hair. At last the final sound of the elevator. It is 7:00 P.M. We are all exhausted by our conversations with the busy people, yet I must find the strength to listen to the elusive neurologist. He talks of some rare metabolic disorder called "Cytochrome C Oxidase Deficiency," and my heart explodes.

Suggestions

- Family choice should be exercised in determining the team of health care providers involved in the care of the child. Minimize anxiety for the family by providing available options before decisions are made and by openly discussing the role of each provider.
- Do not rob the family of their dignity in the process of providing health care to the child. Should it become necessary for the child to receive treatment in a medical teaching environment, the family should not be unnecessarily subjected to repetitive examinations and discussions with providers beyond the medical team for the purpose of "team teaching" medical residents. Resident doctors and other health care providers should be permitted to examine the

child and elicit information from the family only upon prior agreement with the family.

Communication with Families

Communication between the family and the health care provider is one of the cornerstones of family-centered care and is a fundamental opportunity for the provider to establish a collaborative relationship with the family. Since family-centered care is a paradigm shift that requires health care providers to acknowledge the family as an equal partner in meeting the unique health care needs of the child, providers are encouraged to learn new and creative ways of communicating with the family to facilitate this partnership. In a collaborative relationship, both the health care provider and the family must feel comfortable in expressing their honest thoughts and feelings and each must be afforded the opportunity to discuss options openly in a clear and respectful manner.

Since communication is a vital component to building mutual trust and respect with the family, many of the recommendations stated below may appear redundant. However, it is important to expand on their meaning in the context of communication and, in doing so, reiterate their value and importance in creating a collaborative relationship with the family.

- Listen to the family, without preconceived notions or judgments.
- Explain medical terminology in a clear and concise manner.
- Openly share information relevant to the health care of the child in an effort to assist the family in making informed choices.
- Offer medical recommendations as options for the family, and support the family in their decision even if their choice differs from that of the provider.
- Consider differing abilities to understand and process given information.
- Create an environment for open communication by assertively expressing medical recommendations without denying the needs and rights of the family.
- Refer the family to appropriate community resources and services.

Cytochrome C Oxidase Deficiency. There are still few answers to what this means. We have put Michael through test after test and the only thing I know for sure is that there will always be one more doctor who will undoubtedly order yet one more procedure. No one has answers. Everyone is curious. I am beginning to realize that the more accommodating we are as parents, the less information we receive. I can get no written information, biopsy results, or details that will help us better understand what we are dealing with. The "unknowingness" is worse than the disease itself. The busy people only take from us—a piece here, a piece there—leaving us stripped of any dignity or hope for our son. . . .

Michael's fourth birthday. Family and friends are joyful with thanks; doctors are still "cautiously optimistic." Each year we rejoice that he is still with us despite all predictions. He truly is a celebration of life; yet, I am weary of recreating his death in my mind each day. I live in constant fear, pausing each morning as I open the door to his room, certain that this will be the morning I find him without life. I reluctantly select a meaningful gift on his birthday, fearful it will serve as a torturous memory after he is gone. I cry in bookstores as I pass the childhood treasures that we will never share. It is the ultimate fear that keeps me going, fear that I am not doing all that I can to save him—so I block the morbid image from my mind of my son being lowered in the ground, and I continue to search for answers. . . .

Michael loves the piano. We sit and play each day, and for a moment there is some normalcy in our lives. I foolishly dream that, even if he cannot run and play like other children, he will find joy in music. A letter comes. There are several pages, but only one word pierces my heart like a knife. DEAFNESS, the neurologist is saying Michael will probably go deaf. Are we to be robbed of every hope! What is this based on? Have many other children gone deaf from this illness? I need more information, and he has casually stated DEAFNESS as a probability. How I long to talk to another parent going through this same madness! How I long for some statistical information on how, when, and why this is a probability! Another panicked call to Los Angeles. He does not remember stating deafness as a probability. *Does not remember*. I choke back the tears and try to remain composed. I have learned that a mother must remain "professional" and take on the characteristics of the busy people if she is to get information. I cannot risk being shut out if they choose to label me an "emotional parent," but my body stiffens in anger at his words, "Do not worry about deafness." Is that "do not worry" as in, "Michael will die anyway"? Or is it "do not worry" as in, "I made a mistake and deafness is not a possibility." I dare not ask, for I know that—no matter what his answer—it has been stated, and I will forever see the word *deafness* on page two, third line down from the top. The notion of deafness is now added to the already overwhelming number of concerns forever embedded in my mind. He does not know that worry is not an option, but only the reality of my life. . . .

Michael appears to be doing well in spite of the gross motor delays; however, I notice that he is sometimes more alert than others and that his tremors seem to be worse when I feed him specific foods. There are changes in his stool that alarm me. I repeatedly discuss these concerns with my numerous doctors, but no one seems interested beyond their own area of expertise. To them Michael is not a whole child; he is a heart, a brain, a weakened mass of muscle. When I ask for nutritional guidance, I am told that diet will not affect the outcome of Michael's life. I am made to feel like a foolish mother-in-denial who is trying to "cure" her son with home cooking. Please, somebody, listen to me! I know this child. I understand the severity of his illness and the possibility of death, but that doesn't mean I should abandon his basic needs. Quality of life! Doesn't anyone know or care about the quality of his daily life! Everyone seems so concerned about the "big picture" that no one will listen to me about what seems to affect him on a daily basis. My questions are too simplistic and go unanswered. I read everything I can on nutrition and possible causes of malabsorption. Is it possible that Michael has celiac disease? I begin the task of documenting everything Michael eats—to gain proof, hopefully, for my doctors that my concerns are valid.

Suggestions

- Listen to the concerns of the family, and appropriately respond to those concerns. Parents usually have an innate sense about what is best for their child, and they should be valued and respected for their expertise.
- Choose your words carefully. Remember that the manner in which information is given, and the words that are used, will forever burn in the hearts and memory of the family.

Solving Problems and Resolving Conflicts

In a collaborative approach to health care, both the health care provider and the family acknowledge that conflict is a natural part of any relationship. Since by its very nature the medical community is often stressful for both the family and the provider, it is important for both to develop the skills necessary for conflict resolution if the needs of the child are to be met adequately. Family members who feel respected and supported during times of stress and conflict will more willingly reach agreement with the health care provider and ultimately offer less resistance to medical recommendations for the child. Ideally, the provider and the family should each strive for a mutual agreement that will meet the needs of all parties concerned, while simultaneously acknowledging the family's right to make the final decision.

The following recommendations adapted from *Getting to Yes: Negotiating Agreement without Giving In* (Fisher et al., 1981) can be modeled by the health care professional in an attempt to reach mutual agreement with the family:

- Separate the person from the problem. Both parties can agree that they are in disagreement and that each has a right to his or her own opinion.
- Establish interests, goals, and priorities. Determine how each party defines the circumstances, and identify mutual goals and desired outcomes for the well-being of the child.
- Generate options that can achieve a win/win position. Both parties should remain flexible and open to compromise as they explore all options for the child before making a final decision.
- Strive for agreement. Recognize that the family may need more time to consider and review the options before making a final decision.

> The busy people tell us that a muscle biopsy must be done to confirm the diagnosis of Cytochrome C Oxidase Deficiency. We are not as shocked by the news this time. There is a numb acceptance that there will always be yet one more procedure to be done. The Florida neurologist is chilling in his discussion of five alternative diagnoses that may apply to Michael's condition. Again, I am not surprised that he doubts the opinions of those in Los Angeles. Each possibility he describes is more horrendous than the one before. *All* are fatal. There is little hope or compassion in this man's eyes as he dutifully examines my son. How is it possible that a man can so diligently devote his life to saving children and have such a coldness about him? . . .
>
> We prepare for the surgery. There is a research team of doctors in New York who are studying mitochondrial disorders. I have learned to talk of such things and understand that it will take time for cells to grow for the study. They must receive a frozen biopsy. I ask for a detailed explanation of how and when the biopsy will be transported to New York. The heart biopsy taken in Los Angeles was inadvertently defrosted before the appropriate tests could be completed. I do not want another piece of my son to be wasted. My husband offers to personally deliver the frozen biopsy to New York. We are reas-

sured by Dr. Frost that transporting muscle biopsies is standard procedure. I am "cautiously optimistic."

The procedure is done. Another small piece of my son has been taken and replaced with a tormenting memory. I anxiously wait for a call from Dr. Frost. One month passes. Two. Three. Four. Each month I phone his office to see if there is any news. "No, not yet, Mrs. Spano. These things take time. You must be patient." I am patient. I realize there are many other children who need help. Each time the phone rings, my heart stops. I feel as if I'm on *Let's Make a Deal*, waiting for Dr. Frost to tell me which door I have won. Only there is no prize. The result behind Door No. 1 will kill my son; Door No. 2 will perhaps kill him a little faster than the result behind Door No. 3—and so my thoughts go, each day wondering which disease it will be. What will we be facing? This is the worst four months of my life! The house is solemn. Family and friends keep calling to see if we have heard any news. There is no escape to normalcy. Month Five comes and goes. I feel I am going mad with anxiety.

The phone rings. It's Dr. Frost's office. I can't breathe. The woman on the other end says something about needing insurance verification for some lab work to be completed. I am confused by the conversation. This information was given months ago. I question her on the biopsy. She shows no record of any biopsy being sent to New York. What? My mind races. This can't be happening! But it is happening. The biopsy has been sitting in the pathology lab here in Florida all these months we have been waiting. I am devastated and outraged by the incompetence. But I followed up each month—why didn't they? "Not to worry," says Dr. Frost. It will be flown to New York as soon as possible. More waiting.

"Dr. Frost's office calling. Will you hold, please?" The muscle biopsy does not show any significant abnormalities. Michael appears to be normal. Excuse me, did you say "NORMAL"? How is this possible? How did we get from life-threatening disease to normal? I look over at my five-year-old son, who is still unable to lift his frail body to a standing position, and know that "normal" is not an adjective that describes him. "Well, the biopsy was defrosted before it got to New York. All the tests couldn't be completed. The pathologist did not pack it properly. We think we were able to get enough information from the defrosted biopsy"—on and on the story goes. These are excuses. This is not a definitive explanation that reassures me my son is indeed "normal." I am insulted that Dr. Frost thinks I would be comforted by these nonsensical remarks. Somehow I find the courage to express calmly my anger and frustration. My disappointment. Not my pain. I could never express the pain I am feeling at this moment. He does not apologize. He does not take responsibility for his incompetence. Rather, he blames another and tells me my son is normal. I know I will never recover from the agony of this moment or the past six months. A trust has been broken. If only he had been honest with me! Mistakes can be forgiven; dishonesty cannot.

Michael has taught me that, even in the darkest moment, one can find light. Even in deceit, there is opportunity for healing. Today I stop living in fear. Today I stop living my life based on the words of a stranger. There will be no more waiting. No more hoping that the busy people will find an answer. Today I begin a new journey—a journey that will allow me to focus on the quality of Michael's life. Today I allow myself to experience my miracle child with joy. I find hope in the realization that the busy people are not omnipotent. Thank you, Dr. Frost, for shattering the illusion. There is a calmness now as I begin again preparing for the next procedure to be done in Los Angeles.

Suggestions

- Remember that as a health care provider you are working with a child and a family—not a "case." The family will bear lifelong emotional consequences based on the actions demonstrated in resolving issues of conflict.
- Acknowledge the family's right to know the truth, even if the truth is painful in that you do not know the answer or you have made a mistake. Deception only serves to rob the family of any remaining dignity or self-esteem.

HOPE FOR THE FAMILY: THE MIRACLE CHILD

I have stated earlier that the underlying premise of family-centered care is that collaboration between the family and the health care provider is vital to the health and well-being of the child. The examples above have hopefully illustrated what it can mean to the *family* when this premise is demonstrated in the medical community. However, what is ultimately meant by the statement that a collaborative relationship will result in greater outcomes for the *child*?

The answer is simple: In a collaborative relationship, families are afforded the opportunity to take responsibility for their own lives. As family members learn to accept this responsibility and respond to their innate sense of what is best for the child, there is a tremendous sense of fulfillment. This opportunity for empowerment ultimately results in a more sophisticated level of involvement in the care of the child, a renewed sense of hope for the child, and overall greater esteem for the family. It is important to remember that services to the child are of little or no value if the family is lacking in esteem, without hope, and unable to cope with the daily challenges. There is no professional level of expertise that ever has the right to rob the family of that hope. For a family facing the complex challenges of a child with special health care considerations, hope is the only strength.

Health care providers, then, are faced with the dilemma of how to meet the challenge of sharing the hard facts of reality about a child's future possibilities or limitations without destroying the family's hope. Too many of our children have surpassed the limited expectations placed on them for providers ever to believe they have all the answers. Yet, what is hope? For providers, *hope* is a big word that rings of accountability. "If I give the family a sense of hope, am I only going to cause them more pain later on? What if I am wrong?" For family members, *hope* is a little word that serves as a coping mechanism in meeting the day-to-day challenges of rearing a child with special needs. Hope is what gets mom through the 999th visit to the physical therapist. Hope is what makes a dad smile when his five-year-old son finally utters his first word. Hope is what keeps the family alive when a child lost behind dead eyes shows a glimmer of expression at the sound of their voices. The health care provider can meet the challenge of balancing reality with hope if emphasis is placed on the positive attributes of the child and a conscious effort is made to acknowledge the family for the contributions they have made to the successes of that child. The greatest gift we can offer the child is the experience of a whole loving family. *The greatest gift we can offer a family is the opportunity to experience the miracle of their child.*

In conclusion I offer this final personal example as an illustration of how the family has the innate capacity to heal from the loss of the dream child and move to the joyful experience of the miracle child. Family-centered care and the underlying premise of collaboration with the family is an opportunity for the health care provider to support the family in that healing process.

> He is twelve years old now and entering middle school. I have grown somewhat accustomed to the idea of death and no longer fear it. It is still a daily reality for me, but Michael's smile and joyful conversa-

tion shield me from painful thoughts. I am thankful for each day that he is here. Even his adolescent backtalk gives me delight. Until now I have never allowed myself to think beyond the moment, but he is talking of college and things I never dreamt possible. I am no longer pushing him—he is pulling me toward his own greater vision. The world still sees a frail little body disabled by disease as he struggles in his walker, but I do not see the child they see. He is a boy filled with laughter, and I proudly marvel at his gift to enchant everyone he meets with his spirit and his joy of life. He has taught us how to value the simpler things. I am calmer now. It is no longer important to me that he walk, only that he live his life to the fullest. His speech is still not perfect and nothing about him resembles the image of the dream child so long ago imagined. Yet, every day he surprises me with another new word or phrase he has learned; and whatever he is, it is enough. There is a magic about him that is greater than any child of perfection I could ever have created in my mind. He loves to read and is a wiz on the computer. School is his favorite activity. The busy people have given us several more labels throughout the years. Celiac Disease. Hyshimoto's Disease. Too many biopsies have been lost or destroyed for us to rely on the diagnosis of Cytochrome C Oxidase Deficiency with any certainty; yet, it is something we cling to when there is a need to believe we have answers. I still watch to make sure he is hearing that faraway sound. The fear of deafness will never leave me. People gravitate toward him. There is an uncanny zest for adventure about him as though he secretly knows he must grab whatever is out there while he can. We do not talk of death. There is no need for him to know the anguish I have known.

"Mommy, can we go to Japan, London, Chicago, New York?" He watches geography shows on television and judiciously saves his money for travel, wanting to see and do it all. *Planes, Trains, and Automobiles* is his favorite movie. "Wichita?" Maybe we'll skip Wichita, son.

He loves basketball and most of his clothes reflect his admiration for Michael Jordan. He practices shooting baskets from a small chair in his room, never asking why he can't play outside with the other boys. He is a boy, just like any other adolescent boy who challenges his parents' authority one minute and desperately cries, "Mom, I need your help," in the next. There is a wisdom in his eyes and a spirit about him that friends say comes from us. It is difficult for me to know if we have given him strength or he has given it to us. I suspect that we are the receivers. I do know for certain that his experience of life would be very different if we had given up hope and continued to live in fearful agony. We have done all that is humanly possible to give him a joyful childhood in spite of the obstacles. He now struggles for independence in a world that is only beginning to accept that dignity does not have to be lost to disability.

"Mom, can I take karate with the other kids?" Oh, God! Doesn't he know he has a disability? Well, son, karate could be a bit difficult. "That's O.K., Mom. I'll just show the other kids how guys with a disability do it in a wheelchair."

"Mom, can I go to the roller-skating party at school?" Oh, God! This child is wearing me out. Well, roller-skating could be a bit challenging for us, Michael. "Mom, don't worry. If I fall down, you can pick me up again. It's not a big deal, Mom."

We do not talk of his illness as a good or bad thing. There is nothing right or wrong about disability. It just is. Michael understands that he has limitations and that he is different. He is secure in his uniqueness. "Mom, I'm just a little bit 'dipperent,' aren't I? I do things in my own way."

And so it's time for another appointment. This time it's the allergist. The young doctor greets us in the waiting room and is astonished by the frail little boy before him, struggling through the door in his walker. As we talk, clearly Dr. Kindness is overwhelmed by the obvious severity of Michael's condition. Over and over he repeats that he is "just a traditional allergist." We are making him nervous. I calmly begin the recitation of Michael's various illnesses, careful not to overwhelm him with the "big one." I need this man's help, so I must find a way to ease his discomfort. He shyly asks question after question of me, eyes cast downward, careful never to acknowledge Michael's presence in the room. I am not angered by this. I can sense that he is scared. I will help him learn not to fear children who are different. Finally, the million-dollar question: What is the primary diagnosis? I slowly state, "Cytochrome C Oxidase Deficiency," knowing that, like so many other doctors I have met, he will have little understanding of what this means. He has a look of confusion on his face. I open my mouth to explain as Michael gleefully exclaims, "Wow! What a big word! I hope he can spell it." With that, the room fills with laughter. Dr. Kindness relaxes, and I breathe a sigh of relief that Michael has once again led me out of the darkness.

Later, I silently tell myself that maybe, just maybe, I haven't done such a bad job, after all, of creating normalcy in Michael's life. To him the diagnosis that has caused me so much anguish is simply a "big word." It does not reflect his experience of life. He does not live in sorrow or self-pity. He somehow seems to know what it has taken me years to realize: Life is simply what we make of it in our own minds. There are no guarantees, no easy solutions, no way to predict the future. A diagnosis is an educated guess about what we believe to be true at one moment in time. People die who shouldn't. People live when we don't expect them to. There is freedom in acceptance of this innocent knowledge. Perhaps it is Michael's own innocence that has kept him alive beyond all predictions. There is no longer a need to find answers for why he is here or how long he will remain with us. For now, it is enough to know that we are blessed with the miracle of Michael.

REFERENCES

Dunst, C. J. (1991). Implementation of the individualized service plan. In M. J. McGonigel, R. K. Kaufmann, & B. H. Johnson, eds., *Guidelines and recommended practices for the individualized family service plan*, 2nd ed. Bethesda, MD: Association for the Care of Children's Health.

Edelman, L., Greenland, B., & Mills, Bessie L. (1992). *Building parent/professional collaboration*, Project Copernicus Train-the-Trainer Series. St. Paul, MN: Pathfinder Resources.

4

The Challenge of Communication with Parents

Stanley D. Klein

If communicating with parents is a critical aspect of pediatric care, why is it that the training of pediatricians, like the training of colleagues in other pediatric health care disciplines, rarely includes specific content about the doctor–parents relationship or the role of the family in health care (Kerns & Turk, 1985)? Is it assumed that communication skills with parents will develop "naturally" in each clinician, and that neither concepts nor techniques for interacting with parents need to be taught (Wolraich & Reiter, 1979)?

In recent years, while parents of children with disabilities and special health care needs have received increasing attention in clinical education programs such as the ones described in other chapters in this book, such content usually focuses on parental reactions and adaptation so that the student clinician can have a better appreciation of the life of the family. The teaching of specific applications of this knowledge to day-to-day clinical interactions with parents is just beginning to develop.

This chapter presents specific concepts about the health care professional–parent relationship and the communication of information—often called "patient education information"—to parents.[1] My goal is to see the skilled clinician be able to integrate these concepts and techniques into his or her day-to-day work with parents in ways that fit with the individual personal style of the clinician, the demands and constraints of the health care setting in which the professional practices, and the needs of the parents.The first section below will discuss the etiology and treatment of professional attitudes toward parents that can undermine parent–professional collaboration. The second section will concentrate on concepts and techniques that can be applied to the range of parent–professional interactions likely to occur in health care and education settings. A step-by-step process for delivering difficult diagnostic news to parents will be presented in the third section. And in the fourth section, the challenge of teaching these concepts and techniques will be discussed.

ATTITUDES TOWARD PARENTS

Many health care professionals view parents negatively—as nervous, guilty, anxious, depressed, and/or overprotective.[2] Such negative stereotyping probably begins to develop as inexperienced clinicians-in-training observe parents in health care settings. These clinicians seem to ignore the fact that the sample of behavior they observe is not representative of any parent's everyday adaptation to parenting; rather, it is an observation of parts under significant stress brought about by concerns for a child's health and the potentially frightening implications of any health care assessment. Unfortunately, after observing many parents under the stress of seeking health care for a child with a "problem," health care professionals often conclude that *all* parents are anxious, inept, inadequate, troubled adults *all* the time.

In addition to observing parents under the stress of clinical care, most health care professionals have these clinical learning experiences at a developmental stage in their own personal lives (as young adults) during which they are in the process of establishing themselves as independent individuals. It is common for young adults to blame their own perceived inadequacies on their parents' lack of parenting abilities. Thus, the stage-specific "complaints" of young health care professionals in reference to their own "dysfunctional" parents serve to confirm their observations of their young patients' parents. Parenthetically, although I am an advocate for personal psychotherapy, I suspect that young professionals who are participating in psychotherapy may be particularly vulnerable to this skewed sort of observation.

Finally, "pop psychology," as reported by the public media as well as some professional literature, continues to blame parents—especially mothers—for the problems of children and, retrospectively, for the problems of adults—thereby "validating" the personal and clinical experiences of the developing professional. For example, a review of 125 articles in reference to psychological disorders of children found that "mothers are held responsible for 72 different kinds of psychological disorder" (Caplan,

1986, p. 20). Despite increasing research and clinical evidence of the role of constitutional characteristics in the development of both physical and mental illnesses, the stigmatizing of parents continues in professional literature (Seligman & Seligman, 1980). (See Chapter 9 for a discussion of some of the sociological factors that shape physicians' attitudes toward parents.)

The unfortunate result of all these kinds of experiences in the lives of developing health care providers is that many professionals unwittingly bring negative stereotypes (prejudices) into their encounters with parents—which, in turn, interfere with the professionals' perceptions and their ability to communicate constructively with parents (Klein, 1982). Seligman and Darling (1989), in their wonderful book *Ordinary Families, Special Children*, review many studies regarding the negative attitudes of professionals toward parents of children with disabilities, and illustrate the destructive impact of such attitudes.

To counteract actively the factors that create such negative stereotypes and that contribute to the blaming of parents, developing professionals need opportunities to discuss their perceptions and attitudes and to be willing to learn from parents via a variety of teaching formats. These formats can range from parents as lecturers and panelists, to professionals participating in home visits and respite care. In any case, the need to create opportunities like these is imperative. Unless brought to consciousness and addressed, the prejudice against parents may be passed on as clinical wisdom to future generations of health care providers (Seligman & Seligman, 1980).

A far more appropriate perspective on the parents of young patients is to learn to appreciate, first, that parents are the experts about their child and can serve as teachers to professionals (Northcutt, 1980; Cruickshank, Morse & Grant, 1990) and, second, that parents should be partners in the diagnostic and treatment processes. This perspective is clearly articulated in recent federal legislation in the United States, which seeks to establish early intervention and family support programs for families that include an infant or toddler with disability and/or serious medical condition. (See Public Law 99-457, Education of the Handicapped Act Amendment, U.S. Congress, and related regulations prepared by the U.S. Office of Education, 1986; see also Seligman & Darling, 1989; Zambone, 1990.) This perspective has also been articulated by Sia and Peter:

> An important aspect of treating children and families is developing and nurturing the parent–professional relationship. There is a growing movement toward

establishing partnerships between parents and professionals. In this way, parents and professionals can maximize their individual abilities to enhance treatment by forging an alliance that will be beneficial to the overall care for the child.

> Effective parent–professional partnerships are the embodiment of family centered care. Just as family centered care requires that we reevaluate the way we interact with families, the idea of partnership implies a move away from traditional treatment models. (Sia & Peter, 1989, p. 98)

One illustration of parental expertise is in the research demonstrating that, when parents' abilities to assess a child—such as estimating their child's developmental levels in specific areas—have been studied, parents do as well or better than professional "experts" (Vincent, 1988; Schopler & Reichler, 1972). Nonetheless, the concept of parents as experts can be troubling for some clinicians. While the professional expects the parents to provide information, he or she is unlikely to expect parents to take an active role in decision making (Lusthaus, Lusthaus & Gibbs, 1981). Rather, parents may be expected to be passive and cooperative, prepared to agree with professionals (Gliedman & Roth, 1980).

As mentioned above, mothers in particular have been blamed for all sorts of childhood "problems." Historically, rather than being perceived as experts, the mothers of children with disabilities have been misperceived by professionals (mostly males) as hostile and demanding and probably psychopathological. In contrast, more recent literature on female development (Miller, 1976) makes clear that, when women speak out on behalf of the needs of loved ones, they are asserting themselves in a psychologically healthy and appropriate fashion.

The partnership concept is particularly relevant in the care of children with disabilities because many of these children require long-term day-to-day management and care, usually delivered or supervised by parents (Mumford, 1985). In the literature on models of the doctor–patient relationship, the mutual participation model (Szasz & Hollender, 1975) is considered most appropriate for "chronic" conditions because the doctor and the patient (and/or parents) work together toward mutual goals. This collaborative model is likely to be effective when there are common goals, a common understanding of the problem, and a common plan for treatment (Alpert & Wittenberg, 1986). This model is *not* appropriate in acute illness situations in which the doctor tells the patient (or parents) what to do and/or administers the treatment directly to a relatively passive patient (Mumford, 1985).

Studies of patient compliance support the collaborative model, even though the term *compliance* suggests an authoritarian approach by the provider (Billings & Stoeckle, 1989). In a pediatric setting, Korsch and

Negrete (1972) demonstrated that key factors in parental (mothers') cooperation with physicians and in successful health outcomes for children included the following: a mother's perception that the doctor praised her as a mother; an active exchange between doctor and mother; a physician's expression of concern for the mother's feelings; and the mother's satisfaction with the visit. Similarly, in special education settings, Witt et al. (1984) found that parental satisfaction is related to having adequate time, having input from professionals, being involved in the discussion, and not being blamed.

From a practical point of view, this means that the process of meeting the health care needs of a child will be enhanced when the health care professionals believe that the interaction with the child's parents will be one of active reciprocal learning—parents and professionals learning from one another how best to help the child. In his recent book, Greenspan notes, "It should go without saying that the parents are the true integrators of all that relates to the child, as they are with the child the most hours of the day. They not only need to benefit from the insights of all the professionals who work with the child, they need to provide feedback to the professionals about what works and doesn't work at home, as well as the emotional climate there" (1992, pp. 686–687).

It is well known that, in learning, the self-esteem of the learner is critical. In relation to parents, Baker (1980) found that, when parents feel more competent, they become more effective. Therefore, to facilitate learning (and teaching) by parents, the professional needs to demonstrate clearly his or her respect for the expertise of the parents and also needs to acknowledge explicitly their role as active partners.

Brazelton (1988) poignantly illustrated how the professional's approach to a parent can impact parental self-esteem and thereby facilitate participation. He described a situation in which pediatric residents were distressed that the teenage mothers they were seeing in the clinic had no questions to ask after an initial physical examination of their new babies. When the residents followed Dr. Brazelton's suggestion that they begin their contact with a positive comment about the mother and her new baby, the mothers had many questions.

CONCEPTS AND TECHNIQUES FOR COLLABORATION

Setting

It will be assumed here that it is usually important for the health care professional to meet with parents separately from their very young child/

patient (but see below in reference to older children). The setting in which such a discussion of the child's history or of clinical findings occurs should convey a mutual participation model of communication by encouraging an active give-and-take among adults of equal status. Practically speaking, this means that the setting ought to be arranged with the following considerations: (1) all participants should be seated in equally comfortable chairs; (2) each seated adult's eyes must be on the same level as all the others; (3) each must be seated at a conversational distance from the others; and (4) each participant should be able to take notes comfortably (Klein, 1979; Buckman, 1992). And "only if it is absolutely impossible to sit down should you try and hold a significant clinical interview standing" (Buckman, 1992, p. 45).

Accordingly, a separate room (or seating area) with a desk and adult-sized chairs (and a box of tissues) is more appropriate than using an examining room (along with nearby medical equipment) or a classroom or playroom with furniture designed for young children. In addition, parents are entitled to uninterrupted privacy according to a pre-arranged schedule that respects the value of their time as well as the professionals', and that allows sufficient time for discussion along with an opportunity to continue, if necessary, at another time. (See Billings & Stoeckle, 1989, for discussions of similar issues in the doctor–adult patient relationship.)

Once children are ten to twelve years of age, meeting with the parents apart from the children is not likely to be constructive, because it creates the impression that the parents and the professionals are on the same "side" at a time in the child's life when she or he is likely to need the health care professional as a supportive ally or advocate "against" the parents. Since separate meetings also create the impression that the clinician is communicating something different to the parents than to the child, meeting with the parents and the child together—while at the same time providing an opportunity for confidential doctor–patient communication for the child—will be more constructive as long as the professional, by words and by action, focuses attention on the child and the child's health care needs.

Include Dad

Whenever possible, we need to encourage the child's father to participate. All too often, despite the recent cultural awareness of sexism, mother is expected to attend meetings in reference to a child's health or education—as if she were at home with nothing else to do, while her traditional husband's work is too important to be interrupted by such trivial matters! In this same scenario, the mother is expected to report to the father so that he can provide his stamp of approval and pay the bill. In a study of hundreds of individual education planning (IEP) committee meetings regarding special education assessments—meetings to which both parents were invited—both parents were present in only 9 percent of the meetings (Cruickshank, Morse & Grant, 1990).

Involving the father—which may still require a special invitation, to counteract stereotypical male behavior—will communicate the message that he too has an important parenting role. Involving fathers is especially important when parents are expected to carry out or supervise compliance or to participate in a treatment program at home. Even when divorced fathers do not share in child custody, they can participate.

> Traditionally, fathers have not been actively involved in the educational and health care needs of their children. By involving fathers from the start (including fathers who may not be living with their children), clinicians demonstrate to children as well as their parents that fathers are important. It is not unusual for a boy to get the idea, based on his observations of his mother and most of his teachers (usually women), that school is girl's work. At the same time, fathers, when confronted with a child who is awkward and/or somewhat disappointing, are more likely than mothers to withdraw their efforts to be with their son. This unfortunate cycle of disappointment, frustration and withdrawal can be altered by involving fathers from the beginning and letting fathers know just how important they are. Fathers are usually very responsive to this approach, often reporting that it is the first time they have not felt left out by health professionals. (Klein, 1982, pp. 114–115)

Fathers of children with disabilities are beginning to get attention: "Families and professionals now have the chance to build new bridges, to drastically construct a vision that gives fathers of children with disabilities recognition and understanding, and most importantly, substantive programs—not add-ons—that speak to dads' unique concerns" (May, 1992, p. 39).

How Many Professionals?

In some multidisciplinary settings, clinical findings and recommendations are presented to parents at a "team" meeting in which every health care professional involved in the assessment of their child is present and has a turn at presenting the finding in her or her area of specialty. In medical teaching situations, the "entourage" may also attend.

Some school systems convene similar mass meetings when the special education assessment of a child is completed, because it is erroneously believed that the federal law regarding special education and related services mandates such meetings. In fact, the federal law actually states that three professionals must attend every meeting with parents at which individualized education plans are created. Cruickshank, Morse, and Grant (1990) found that an average of five professionals attended, and sometimes as many as ten to twelve attended. Greater numbers were usually related to greater severity of a child's disability.

Most parents report feeling overwhelmed when the number of professionals exceeds the number of parents! And many professionals believe that those meetings involving all the professionals tend to contribute to a fragmented approach to the child and family, rather than the integrated approach such meetings are supposed to facilitate.

For most parents, smaller meetings with one or two key professionals are preferable. One of the professionals present should be prepared to be the person involved in follow-up communications. Some parents find the participation of a trained parent advocate very helpful (Klein, 1979).

Planning and Preparation

Whenever possible, it is helpful for professionals to communicate with parents in advance (in person, by telephone, or by mail) about structural details such as the meeting time (both starting time and finishing time, the meeting place (how to get there, where to park, etc.), the names and functions of all participants, and the agenda. Parents can also be invited to modify the agenda.

The professional team needs to prepare itself for meetings with parents. All such meetings require thoughtful preparation; the more professionals in attendance, the more complicated the planning process becomes. One person needs to be identified as the leader—the person who will assume responsibility for introducing (or reintroducing) each team member to the parents, for keeping the meeting focused on the agenda, and for appropriate follow-up with the family. The team needs to agree on the key messages they wish to convey and should prepare how to present them so that the meeting can proceed without anyone's being rushed. Ideally, the team can also learn to model such interpersonal skills as attentive listening, mutual support, respectful give-and-take, and the ability to help one another communicate clearly (Klein, 1979).

Creating the Parent–Professional "Partnership"

Since parents may have served only as informants in prior relationships with health care providers, the importance of their active participation as observers and experts will need to be stated early in the process—such as during the developmental history. In those situations when parents have already provided a developmental history to another provider or at another setting, it is helpful to apologize for the repetitiousness and to explain the purpose of a case history in the current context. In addition, to counteract the common parental experience that a case history is like a courtroom interrogation in which parents are on trial, the health care professional can make clear that the parents are not being judged on the basis of whatever they did or did not do, and that it is unrealistic to expect parents to remember every developmental detail for every child. Parents need to hear that they are not being blamed for their actions or criticized for forgetting historical data. Rather, one purpose of the discussion is for parents to share their observations as well as their questions and concerns.

Another technique for addressing parental worries about being judged is for the health care professional to demonstrate explicitly his or her *empathy* with the parents by acknowledging that parenting is always difficult and that parenting a child with a disability can result in parents' feeling upset, frustrated, angry, and/or discouraged (other human feelings also being possible). Similarly, the clinician can clarify in a supportive manner that the parents would probably like to enjoy their parenting more (Greenspan, 1992). Via such specific empathic comments, the clinician conveys an understanding of parental dilemmas and addresses the common complaint of many parents that health care providers do not really appreciate the day-to-day challenges of caring for children with disabilities and/or special health care needs. (For a discussion of empathy and understanding, see Bernstein & Bernstein, 1985; see also Korsch & Negrete, 1972; Klein, 1979, 1982; Selig, 1983.)

By acknowledging the "negative" feelings that parents experience, the clinician also helps the parents become more active, because in the doctor's office many parents believe they are expected to be "mature," "objective," and stoic.

To do this, parents are likely to suppress their feelings of frustration and worry. This process takes a great deal of psychic energy which is then unavailable for active participation in the diagnostic process. The clinician begins the process of freeing up this energy and thereby facilitating communication and understanding by providing parents with an opportunity to talk about their feelings and by responding with empathy and attention rather than with implied or explicit criticism, or impatience to get on with the procedures.

The clinician's goal is not to cure parents of their frustrations. Rather, as parents have an opportunity to express their feelings to the doctor and to each other, new energy for the task at hand becomes available, energy previously expended on keeping these feelings hidden. In a sense, the parents' emotional block to talking and learning is being treated. During such discussions, parents need to be assured that they are the most valuable people in their child's life and that they can be invaluable in all efforts on behalf of their child. (Klein, 1982, p. 116)

Another useful technique for actively involving parents is to inquire about the *parents' observations* of the child's development—observed in their everyday interactions—in areas relevant to the particular health concerns (such as hearing, language, motor skills, memory, intelligence, reading, social skills, etc.) that the clinician will be objectively and subjectively assessing during the examination. This process also enables the professional to explore parental expectations in relation to the child's "problems" and their remediation, and it sets the stage for connecting parental observations with specific clinical findings following the examination of the child (Alpert & Wittenberg, 1986; Klein, 1982; Klein & Klein, 1987). By linking parental observations to clinical findings, the establishment of shared treatment priorities by the parent–professional "partnership" is facilitated.

In discussing clinical findings, health care professionals need to speak in *understandable language*. Few parents, including well-educated people, understand technical medical and educational terminology. Professionals tend to overestimate the level of understanding of adults. For example, Alpert and Wittenberg (1986) found that adult patients actually understood only twenty-nine of the fifty medical terms that their physicians had thought appropriate for conversations with them.

When treatment priorities require parental involvement with their child in a *program at home*, the mutual participation or partnership model can help prevent the professional team from establishing unrealistic expectations likely to lead to noncompliance. For example, although a particular home-therapy program may ideally require thirty minutes a day from a parent and a child working together, the professional can review how much time is actually available within the constraints of everyday family life and begin with smaller, more realistic increments of time. In this way, both the child and the parents can begin the process by feeling successful, rather than feeling inadequate to the task. Gradually, the "partners" can decide to increase the demands (Klein, 1982).

DELIVERING DIFFICULT NEWS

In the video *Breaking the News* (Institute for Families of Blind Children, 1991), ophthalmologists discuss their feelings and experiences when conveying a serious diagnosis to parents.[3] (Information about obtaining this video is included in the Resource Appendix at the end of the book.)

> When you have to tell a parent the bad news, it's probably one of the most important parts of our job as a physician. . . . It's just unfortunate, we are the least prepared for that aspect. . . . I wish I had a cheat sheet—a step by step, here's the way you do it. (Kenneth W. Wright, M.D., on camera in Institute for Families of Blind Children, 1991)

> We are detached from the impact on parents. . . . I've seen physicians say, "Get used to it. Come to grips with it." . . . I've seen doctors not even tell, not even approach the parents . . . send in one of their trainees. (William V. Good, M.D., on camera in Institute for Families of Blind Children, 1991)

Communicating clinical findings that indicate a child has a serious medical problem and/or developmental disability is a challenging parent-education responsibility. There is no way any practitioner can make the sad news about cerebral palsy, mental retardation, or cystic fibrosis sound like good news (Alpert & Wittenberg, 1986): "Unfortunately, there can be no anesthetic that removes the pain of bad news" (Buckman, 1992, p. 18).

Instead, the professional can have the significant clinical goal of providing parents with an opportunity to begin to mourn the loss of the healthy "perfect" child they may have anticipated, and can facilitate the parents' active participation in their unique parenting (Golden, 1979; Solnit & Start, 1961; Wolff & Simons, 1985). In this way, the clinician can continue to be "a healer despite his failure [to maintain health]. . . . He can initiate the healing process in the patient's deep psychological wound" (Cholden, 1958, p. 29).

One reason the task of delivering "bad" news can be especially difficult for a health care clinician is that it contrasts so dramatically with health care situations that the practitioner finds gratifying—for example, successfully treating an acute medical crisis (Fitzgerald, 1973; Wabrek, 1986).

> You have been trained how to deal with certain things, situations . . . you know what to do; you feel comfortable. We are really not trained to take care of the situation where there is nothing to do . . . very uncomfortable situation. (Kenneth W. Wright, M.D., on camera in Institute for Families of Blind Children, 1991)

In the difficult-news situation, the doctor—as well as the parents—can experience the situation as a tragedy. This is especially likely when there is little that the provider can do to improve immediately the child's condition. It is helpful for the clinician to appreciate his or her own feelings of frustration, disappointment, helplessness, failure, and sadness when unable to do what he or she likes to do best (Solnit & Stark, 1961).

When unable to "fix" the problem, the clinician may erroneously believe that there is nothing that he or she, as a health care practitioner, can do to help the family or the child (Wolff & Simons, 1985). This is an unfortunate error because, even as parents are faced with the inevitability of a child's terminal illness, there is a great deal that the practitioner can do to help the child, parents, and other family members: "Helping patients deal with loss is one of the most difficult and delicate tasks we face . . . all the more so because our training places a premium on 'doing something to the patient' rather than talking or listening. Emotion is discouraged in favor of scientific objectivity" (Wabrek, 1986, p. 88).

For some professionals—particularly some medical subspecialists and clinicians at diagnostic centers—delivering sad news to parents can be an everyday, relatively routine task. In dramatic contrast, for individual sets of parents, hearing the news for the first time will be an experience that will never be forgotten—"a significant event that may alter their lives forever" (Sia & Peter, 1989, p. 93). Etched in the parents' memories and painfully reviewed again and again in the years to come, this first encounter will influence parental perceptions of professionals in the future—sometimes in irreparable ways.

> Be aware of the unique dramatic nature of the diagnostic meeting. Families will remember the moment in which it was presented. You may have diagnosed this condition many times, but for the individual it is a unique historical moment. (Healy & Lewis-Beck, cited in Sia & Peter, 1989, p. 88)

> What the doctor does will affect the parents for the rest of their lives. (A. Linn Murphee, M.D., on camera in Institute for Families of Blind Children, 1991)

Other factors involved in professionals' difficulty with "breaking bad news" are discussed in Chapter 9.

Because of the magnitude of the impact this encounter can have on parents, professionals must approach the challenge with sensitivity and appreciate that the process will take time. It cannot be carried out in a constructive fashion when the bad news is presented by a professional standing with his or her hand on the doorknob, poised to go on to the next "case." Rather, it requires a time-consuming, step-by-step discussion, with everyone seated.

It is crucial to acknowledge that some professionals are unable to set aside sufficient time to be with the parents for this difficult interaction; others do not feel up to the task, temperamentally. Under such circumstances, the parents will need a capable substitute who is prepared to take charge of communicating the findings on behalf of the clinical team.

Starting during the Case History

The time to prepare for the presentation of difficult news is while reviewing the case history with the parents. Ordinarily, during the case-history session, the clinician can quickly gauge the probability that the child has a serious problem. Not only is it important to explore parents' ideas about the etiology of various symptoms so as to recognize the level of their expertise; the case-history session also provides information about the parents' understanding of the body and how it works, and enables the clinician to be prepared to correct misconceptions later on.

Step-by-Step Presentation

The news will be upsetting no matter how it is presented. However, the practitioner can present the clinical findings in a thoughtful step-by-step manner that takes into account the parents' predictable shock and distress and that provides appropriate patient-education information (Alpert & Wittenberg, 1986).

By beginning with a review of the parents' observations and concerns already voiced during the case history, followed by the clinician's own observations that confirm or further clarify those of the parents, the clinician can gradually move to the diagnosis and prognosis. For example, when a one-year-old infant has cerebral palsy and a hearing impairment, the clinician can review the parents' observations about the child's delayed motor development and/or apparent inattentiveness. He or she can then describe examination findings that support the parents' own observations. After that, clinical findings such as reflex abnormalities and electroencephalography results, which go beyond the parents' observations, can be described to explain the internal system conditions that cause the child's observable behaviors.

The principle of patient education here is that the clinician begins with externally observable behaviors and then takes the parents "inside" the child's body and explains in lay terms the relationships between internal processes and observable behaviors—without using the specific diagnostic terminology. The reason for not yet using the specific diagnostic term is to maintain the parents' attention while linking parental observations with clinical findings.

Then the clinician must present the specific news in the form of technical diagnostic terminology. Some practitioners may want to "protect" parents from the pain and distress likely to be associated with the diagnostic terminology. As a result, they may communicate via euphemisms or postpone using the clinical terminology (Borish, 1975; Darling, 1979; Haan, 1979; Sia & Peter, 1989). However, since the parents are usually aware that something is amiss and are worried about it, the practitioner's avoidance of direct discussion is not helpful: It leaves parents fearful and uncertain.

More specifically, without the clinical diagnostic terminology, parents are cut off from three valuable sources of information—information that can empower parents to learn and to grow. First, the clinician who speaks openly about diagnosis can more easily discuss the possible future problems and how to cope with them (Kleinstein & Stone, 1978). Second, informed parents will be able to educate themselves via parent-education materials that are categorized by diagnostic terms. Third, since local and national parent support groups are usually organized according to specific diagnoses, parents without diagnostic information cannot network with other parents with similar children and benefit from the emotional support and information so essential to adaptation.

Once parents have heard the diagnosis, the clinician must take the time to explore the parents' reaction, their worries and fears. Diagnostic terminology is loaded with emotion and mystery. Professionals need to listen to parental worries about the terminology and take time to explain the meaning of the terminology for the specific child being discussed.

Parental Distress

When faced with the information that his or her child has a disability or serious illness, the average, mature, mentally healthy parent will be very upset. Distress is an understandable, healthy reaction. In his excellent book *How to Break Bad News: A Guide for Health Professionals*, Buckman explains that, when an individual receives bad news, "the range of normal reactions is wide"; and he cautions health care professionals to avoid the temptation to assess responses as "either normal or pathological" (1992, p. 98). Buckman also reminds clinicians to remember that "human beings can experience several emotions simultaneously" (1992, p. 111).

Unfortunately, some parents and some clinicians may feel that parents' emotional distress, fears, and concerns about the future are not relevant subject matter for the doctor–parents encounter. Parents and/or the doctor may believe that the "healthy" way for parents to react is to suppress feelings and act in a stoic fashion.

As described earlier, when any human being suppresses fears and distress, a great deal of psychic energy is consumed (Bernstein & Bernstein, 1985). A parent who is working hard to keep feelings and worries inside has very little energy available to pay attention, listen, and learn the vital information about his or her child's condition that the health care professional can provide. Instead, the practitioner now faces a parent with a temporary "learning disability" caused by emotional stress. Because the parent is upset and preoccupied with inner distress in regard to the child's diagnosis, he or she is unable to learn whatever the clinician wants to teach. A valuable technique at this stage is to say to the parents, " 'Cerebral palsy' is a frightening term." A statement of this kind provides explicit permission for the parents to be frightened. It communicates to parents the message that it is a normal human reaction to be frightened by technical terminology, and especially terminology that suggests their child has a serious problem (Henkind, 1983). Without explicit permission and encouragement, a parent may feel embarrassed by the way he or she feels, silently suppress the feelings, and pretend to understand the doctor's educational presentation when, in fact, he or she is unable to pay attention (Klein & Klein, 1987).

This critical step of acknowledging parents' probable reactions gives parents the opportunity to talk about their shock, fears, sadness, and even anger at the clinician for providing the diagnosis. Parents need a chance to voice their fears, worries, and questions to a clinician who conveys that it is acceptable to be upset and to say so. This enables parents to begin the emotional reaction to loss: the mourning process.

> For most sad patients, you accomplish a major therapeutic act by simply allowing the patient to release feelings. . . . [Y]ou fulfill your professional role by simply providing a setting in which the patient can comfortably express and reflect. (Billings & Stoeckle, 1989, p. 175)

It is important to keep in mind that parents' upset, confusion, anger, and/or questioning behavior (such as questioning the doctor's competence, and repetitive questions about the diagnosis itself) are all manifestations of anxiety—part of the mourning process—rather than hostility.

Accordingly, it is productive for the clinician to say, "I can appreciate how frightening it is to hear this news about your child." Or to say, "I can appreciate that you must have all kinds of feelings, including very angry feelings about getting this news."

Here let me be repetitious for the sake of emphasis. By her or his empathic comments, the clinician explicitly informs parents that strong feelings are permissible and acceptable; the clinician validates parental emotions. Parents need to hear that, under the circumstances, it is normal to have many troubling feelings at the same time—fear, sadness, anger, hopelessness. Parents also need to know that the practitioner is willing to listen patiently and will not criticize any emotional reactions (Kleinstein & Stone, 1978). After the parents describe their feelings, the clinician can gradually provide the educational information that the parents need to understand the diagnosis, to reduce the level of distress, and to begin to carry out proper action to meet the needs of the child and family (Bernstein & Bernstein, 1985).

By encouraging parents to discuss their emotional reactions, the clinician helps parents begin to mourn (Wabrek, 1986). It is helpful to explain to parents that they are likely to experience a wide range of emotions because they will be going through the mourning process—mourning the loss of the healthy child of their dreams (Solnit & Stark, 1961). At the same time, by manner and words the clinician communicates that "I will stay with you and, over time, help you learn everything you can to facilitate your parenting." The phrase *over time* is critical, as the mourning process does take time. Giving lip service to a mourning process does not bring it to an end. It will take time—time during which parents will need continued attention and concern, preferably from the clinician who delivered the sad news (Klein & Klein, 1987).

> Once the physician has conveyed the initial diagnosis to the parents there is a tendency to think the interpretation of mental retardation is completed when it has only begun. The main reason for this misconception by the physician is that he has not understood the repetitive aspect of the mourning process . . . their need for repeated opportunities to review. (Solnit & Stark, 1961, pp. 530–531)

While an understanding of stage theory in relation to mourning by parents of children with disabilities can be helpful, some professionals oversimplify the process of mourning by expecting parents to complete all the stages in the "prescribed order" within a short period of time. As Buckman (1992) points out: "human beings do not experience emotions in serial stages, but have their own mixtures of emotions together and simultaneously" (p. 34). Similarly, Seligman and Darling (1989) urge care and caution in the application of stages of mourning to all families (pp. 86–88). The clinician should be guided by a family's reaction rather than assuming a universal need for mourning.

Highly trained health care professionals dedicated to improving health and addressing acute health care needs may have a difficult time with the approach described above, and especially with parents who are upset. Often, talented professionals can perceive the parents' distress and feel upset themselves by the magnitude of the parents' situation. As a result, they cope with their own personal discomfort—and believe they are meeting the need for information—by immediately presenting a thoughtful "lecture" to the parents about the diagnosis and prognosis. In this way, a professional is likely to feel better because he or she is in control and is reassured by his or her expertise. Such behavior is noted by Dr. Christenson: "We get very clinical when we get nervous" (Laurie Christenson, M.D., on camera in Institute for Families of Blind Children, 1991). The clinician may also assume that, as a result of the valuable information conveyed, the parents will understand the child's condition and feel better as well. Instead, the parents suffer quietly, and say little—even when asked whether they have "any questions." They feel embarrassed about being upset—and further embarrassed for failing to understand the "lecture." Surely, parents need a great deal of information; the issue for the clinician is the dosage and timing of information (Klein & Klein, 1987).

Parental questioning can sometimes provoke unproductive clinician behavior, especially when the clinician is uncertain how to respond because the answer is unclear or unknown. Once the professional has first acknowledged the concern expressed by the question, it is appropriate to say "I don't know" or "I'm not sure"—and then to suggest how they both—parents and professionals, as partners—can try to find an answer.

Denial and Anger

Some clinicians have suggested that denial is part of the mourning process; denial is a reaction to anxiety. If a clinician keeps pushing to make a point that a parent denies, the parent's anxiety will increase—further increasing the denial. A more effective technique is to address the cause of the denial itself by talking more with the parents about how frightening and upsetting the bad news can be. Since denial can be considered adaptive as any individual struggles to take in frightening, potentially overwhelming information (Buckman, 1992), there is no immediate need to challenge it.

By specifically encouraging a parent to talk about his or her feelings of anger at the difficult news, the professional helps prevent the clinical depression that can occur in parents as they try to cope with the birth or the initial diagnosis of a child with a disability or serious medical condition (Emerson, 1981). Depression can be the result of a process beginning in angry feelings that are turned inward because there is no opportunity to express the feelings outwardly (Freud, 1957). By addressing parents' feelings, the clinician also has an opportunity to help parents regain their self-esteem and thereby help them remain active participants and learners in the education process.

The professional can also help the parents by explaining the value of verbalizing to one another the wide range of intense feelings each parent is likely to experience in the months to come—including the feeling of "going crazy." Parents need to know that experiencing such feelings is normal and that it is in their own best interest to be able to speak openly about their reactions with their loved ones, as well as with caring professionals. At the same time, as a way of preparing parents to be understanding and supportive of each other, it also can be helpful for parents to be reminded that individuals in mourning can severely test the patience of loved ones by behaving or speaking in troubling ways.

Touching

Although some advocate physical touch as a technique for comforting parents (patients), I suggest caution in this for three reasons. First, it is unlikely that a clinician will be cognizant of specific familial and cultural styles and meanings in relation to touch. Second, since inappropriate touching by psychotherapists, physicians, clergy, and other authority figures has received a great deal of publicity recently, I believe that touch in a clinical setting is now far more likely to be misinterpreted. Third, more and more clinical literature indicates that many adults have been physically and/or sexually abused and, therefore, may be particularly sensitive to even well-intentioned touching. Instead, I suggest that comforting actions be put into words; empathic language can "reach out" in very meaningful ways.

Information Dosages

In discussions on the process of sharing difficult news, many clinicians wonder exactly how much specific detailed information should be conveyed, especially during the stress of first breaking the news. Since little attention has been devoted to this process until recently, I am not aware of any "prescriptions" of information dosages for specific diagnostic conditions. Rather, it seems more useful to appreciate that parental needs for information are likely to change as the child and parents confront different challenges in different settings and reach different stages in their lives.

At the same time, Buckman (1992) offers helpful guidelines in his detailed description of a six-step protocol for breaking bad news. In reference to sharing the information (the fourth of the six steps), Buckman urges a careful presentation of the diagnosis, treatment plan, prognosis, and support and "small chunks," in "English not Medspeak," and with frequent checking of reception. The sixth step includes carefully planning for follow-through and continued support. (See Buckman, 1992, esp. chap. 4, "Breaking Bad News: A Six-step Protocol.")

Many parents of children with disabilities and/or special health care needs hear the diagnostic news for the first time at a referral center, from professionals who will not be directly involved in treatment and long-term care. In such situations, it is essential that the primary care professional (or team) be provided with as much information as possible about the interaction between the parents and the professionals during presentation of the diagnostic news so that the primary care clinician can be prepared to provide for continuing parental needs for support and information.

Support Groups

The professional team also has the responsibility of explaining that parent support groups can provide emotional support and practical information very effectively, often far more effectively than any professional. By becoming participants in such groups, parents no longer feel isolated, can share their grief, and learn practical solutions to everyday challenges.

In order to connect parents with this resource, professionals need to be knowledgeable about the appropriate local and national groups. (Each year, in its September issue, *Exceptional Parent* magazine provides names, addresses, and telephone numbers of all known national parent organizations, listed by diagnostic condition.) However, as experienced parents have pointed out (Greer, 1987), professionals may be asking too much when they expect upset parents of a newly diagnosed child to have the energy and courage to contact a group. Rather, with parental permission, the team can have the group reach out to the "new" parents. In any case, professionals should exercise some caution in referring families to support groups. Although almost all parents need support, some are able to get that support in other ways (e.g., from family or friends) and may not be comfortable with—or may not need—an organized group.

Written Reports

Under the best of circumstances, well-intentioned and intelligent parents are unlikely to remember everything communicated verbally by the health care professional (Alpert & Wittenberg, 1986). While encouraging parents to take notes or to tape-record meetings can be a helpful suggestion, a more effective approach is to explain that it can be very difficult to remember all that has been discussed (Buckman, 1992) and then to prepare a written report for the parents—using language understandable to laypersons—that summarizes the discussion in the meeting, including the clinical findings, the diagnosis, and specific recommendations for treatment and follow-up. Besides helping parents (and clinicians) remember the discussion and thereby prevent the normal distortions in memory that occur over time, such reports can often be valuable for other professionals unfamiliar with the discipline-specific technical language used when professions report to their colleagues.

TRAINING

Although it has been said that "the ability to deal with and communicate bad news . . . should be studied, practiced, and critiqued no less than the more technical skills" (Alpert & Wittenberg, 1986, p. 172) and that it is "essential for professionals in any health care discipline to be as thoroughly trained in patient communication skills as they are in other clinical skills" (Buckman, 1992, p. 23), few health care settings actually provide opportunities for systematic practicing of oral or written communication skills. While meeting parents and interacting with them in a classroom or clinical seminar is valuable because it can affect the professionals' developing attitudes about parents, there is no substitute for learning specific communication techniques.

Student clinicians will also benefit from interacting with adults with disabilities, who can provide real-life examples of "outcomes." Just as professionals' attitudes about parents may be based on negative stereotypes, their discussions with parents about the future for a child may be based on negative stereotypes about the adult lives of people with disabilities or chronic illnesses (Rousso, 1992).

Actors and Actresses

I have used professional as well as well-trained amateur actors and actresses playing parents in order to provide practice, instant replays, and immediate feedback to student clinicians. Individual students are videotaped delivering bad news to actor/patients and then the tapes are reviewed and critiqued in small group discussions. People with acting training are likely to be uniquely perceptive about the details of an interpersonal encounter, and able to respond to content as well as process.

"Dosage" and Sequence

Discussing the proper dosage of information and the best sequence in which to present it is another useful training exercise. Trainees need to sort out the information considered crucial and determine how to present it in a thoughtful, understandable manner. They may need to be reminded that the "lecture" method is not the most useful format for "teaching."

Writing Skills

Writing to educate parents (or patients) also requires practice. While students are often required to write referral letters to colleagues or clinical reports for medical records, I am not familiar with any specific efforts to train professionals to write for parents. My observations, based on requiring students to write letters to patients they have "seen" via video, indicate that some well-educated students have learned to write very complicated, lengthy sentences and paragraphs that are difficult to comprehend. While modern word-processing technology can facilitate efficient report writing, I am very concerned about the need to teach professionals how to present their knowledge in understandable language.

Modeling

Finally, one of our greatest challenges for training is to appreciate the powerful messages conveyed by modeling in the clinical setting. In the current health care context—with many external factors that can detract from good care—each of us can try to maintain high quality care and understanding for parents and be as clear as we can to our students about the compromises we may make.

CONCLUSION

I have presented teachable concepts and techniques for communicating with parents. Unfortunately, selling the need to teach and practice such content continues to be an uphill struggle.

To close, I want to share a list written by a parent about what parents need from professionals (Golden, 1980)—a list of principles that we can try to teach.

- A supportive relationship over time that allows for changing needs, strengths, and external realities as well as recurrent feelings of helplessness and not-knowing.
- A wide view—but one that is also concrete and focused and provides information and tools (practical and emotional) to make the immediate more workable and the future more predictable.
- Validation for correct feelings along with the recognition and assurance that they will not always be the same.
- Respect for a parent's courage to experience and withstand enormous fears, pressures, and unknowns, however these are being expressed.
- Willingness on the part of the professional to find out and not assume or label where a parent is at.
- Help in sorting out the feelings and fears about how things will be from the facts or possibilities, which may be fuller or different.
- Help with (and ongoing reworking of) hopes and expectations that is both challenging and supportive—grounded in reality, yet with room left for feelings and dreams.

NOTES

1. The work on this chapter was supported, in part, by a donation made to Children's Hospital in Boston by Thomas and Barbara Lee.
2. The material in this and the following two sections is adapted from Klein (1982).
3. The material in this section is adapted from Klein and Klein (1987).

REFERENCES

Alpert, J. S., & Wittenberg, S. M. (1986). *A clinician's companion: A study guide for effective and human patient care*. Boston: Little, Brown.

Baker, B. L. (1984). Training parents as teachers of their developmentally disabled children. In S. Salzinger, J. Antrobus & J. Glick, eds., *The ecosystem of the sick child*. New York: Academic Press.

Bernstein, L., & Bernstein, R. S. (1985). *Interviewing: A guide for health professionals*, 4th ed. Norwalk, CT: Appleton-Century-Crofts.

Billings, J. A., & Stoeckle, J. D. (1989). *The clinical encounter: A guide to the medical interview and case presentation*. Chicago: Year Book Medical Publishers.

Borish, I. M. (1975). Breaking the news about cataract. *Optometry Management* 11:13–18.

Brazelton, T. B. (1986). Personal communication.

Buckman, R. (1992). *How to break bad news: A guide for health care professionals*. Baltimore: Johns Hopkins University Press.

Caplan, S. (1986). Blaming Mother. *Psychology Today* 20:10, 20–25.

Cholden, L. S. (1958). Psychiatric aspects of informing the patient of blindness. In L. S. Cholden, *A psychiatrist works with blindness*. New York: American Foundation for the Blind.

Cruickshank, W. M., Morse, W. C., & Grant, J. O. (1990). *The individual education planning committee: A step in the history of special education*. Ann Arbor: University of Michigan Press.

Darling, R. B. (1979). *Families against society: A study of reactions to children with birth defects*. Beverly Hills, CA: Sage.

Emerson, D. L. (1981). Facing loss of vision: The response of adults to visual impairment. *Journal of Visual Impairment and Blindness* 75:41–45.

Fitzgerald, R. G. (1973). The newly blind: Mental distress, somatic illness, disability and management. *Eye, Ear, Nose and Throat Monographs* 52:35–38.

Freud, S. (1957). Mourning and melancholia (1917). In *The standard edition of the complete psychological works of Sigmund Freud*, Vol. 14. London: Hogarth Press.

Gliedman, J., & Roth, W. (1980). *The unexpected minority*. New York: Harcourt Brace Jovanovich.

Golden, S. (1979). Grieving and sharing. *Exceptional Parent* 9:6, C21–C22.

Golden, S. (1980, November). Handout. Boston Institute for the Development of Infants and Parents, Annual Symposium.

Greenspan, S. I. (1992). *Infancy and early childhood: The practice of clinical assessment and intervention with emotional and developmental challenges*. Madison, CT: International Universities Press.

Greer, M. (1987). Personal communications.

Haan, N. G. (1979). Psychosocial meaning of unfavorable medical forecasts. In G. C. Stone, F. Cohen, N. E. Adler, et al., *Health psychology: A Handbook*. San Francisco: Jossey-Bass.

Henkind, P. (1983). Word wounds. *Ophthalmology* 90:31A.

Institute for Families of Blind Children. (1991). *Breaking the news*. Videotape. Los Angeles: Institute for Families of Blind Children. (Information about obtaining this video is included in the Resource List at the end of the book.)

Kerns, R. D., & Turk, D. C. (1985). Behavioral medicine and the family: Historical perspectives and future directions. In D. C. Turk & R. D. Kerns, *Health, illness and families: A life-span perspective*. New York: John Wiley & Sons.

Klein, S. D. (1979). Parent–school conference: Guidelines and objectives. *Exceptional Parent* 9:E19–E21.

Klein, S. D. (1982). The role of the family in helping the child with learning disabilities. In M. Davis and J. C. Whitener, *The role of vision in multi-disciplinary approaches to children with learning disabilities*. Springfield, IL: Charles C. Thomas.

Klein, S. D. (in press). Working with parents: Concepts and techniques. In N. A. S. Barnard & D. F. Edgar, *Paediatric Optometry*. London: Oxford University Press.

Klein, S. D., & Klein, R. E. (1987). Delivering bad news: The most challenging task in patient education. *Journal of the American Optometric Association* 9:660–663.

Kleinstein, R., & Stone, G. (1978). Helping patients to follow their treatment plans. *Journal of the American Optometric Association* 49:1144–1146.

Korsch, B., & Negrete, V. (1972). Doctor–patient communication. *Scientific American* 66:227–230.

Lusthaus, C., Lusthaus, E., & Gibbs, H. (1981). Parents' role in the decision process. *Exceptional Children* 48:256–285.

May, J. (1992). New horizons for fathers of children with disabilities. *Exceptional Parent* 22:3, 40–43.

Miller, J. B. (1976). *The new psychology of women*. Boston: Beacon Press.

Mumford, E. (1985). The responses of patients to medical advice. In R. C. Simons, *Understanding human behavior in health and illness*, 3rd ed. Baltimore: Williams & Wilkins.

Northcutt, W. H. (1980). On behalf of parents in the IEP process. *Volta Review* 82:7–13.

Rousso, H. (1992). Personal communication.

Schopler, E., & Reichler, R. (1972). How well do parents understand their own psychotic child? *Journal of Autism and Childhood Schizophrenia* 2:387–400.

Selig, A. L. (1983). Common myths of family feedback conferences. *Developmental and Behavioral Pediatrics* 4:67–69.

Seligman, M., & Darling, R. B. (1989). *Ordinary families, special children: A systems approach to childhood disability*. New York: Guilford Press.

Seligman, M., & Seligman, P. A. (1980). The professional's dilemma: Learning to work with parents. *Exceptional Parent* 10:S11–S13.

Sia, C., & Peter, M. I. (1989). *The practicing pediatrician and the new morbidity*. Honolulu: Hawaii Medical Association.

Solnit, A. J., & Stark, M. H. (1961). Mourning and the birth of a defective child. *Psychoanalytic Study of the Child* 16:523–537.

Szasz, T. S., & Hollender, M. H. (1956). A contribution to the philosophy of medicine: The basic models of the doctor–patient relationship. *AMA Archives of Internal Medicine* 97:5585–5592.

Vincent, L. J. (1988). What we have learned from families. *OSERS News in Print* 1:3.

Wabrek, A. J. (1986). Help your patient deal with loss. *Med. Econ.* 64:11, 88–93.

Witt, J. E., et al. (1984). Effects of variables on parent perceptions of staffing. *Exceptional Children* 51:27–32.

Wolff, C. T., & Simons, R. C. (1985). Loss, grief, and mourning in adults. In R. C. Simons, *Understanding human behavior in health and illness*, 3rd ed. Baltimore: Williams & Wilkins.

Wolraich, M. L., & Reiter, S. (1979). Training physicians in communication skills. *Developmental Medicine and Child Neurology* 21:773–778.

Zambone, A. M. (1990). Optometrists on the team: Holistic care and patient–parent–educator interface. In A. A. Rosenbloom & M. W. Morgan, *Principles and practice of pediatric optometry*. Philadelphia: J. B. Lippincott.

Part II

Models of Health Provider Education

PRESERVICE MODELS

5

A First-year Medical Student Curriculum about Family Views of Chronic and Disabling Conditions

Judy Lewis
and
Robert M. Greenstein

> I was uncertain about working with a child with Down syndrome. I did not have any experience working with retarded children and really had no concept about his level of functioning or Down syndrome as a "chronic illness." . . . My relationship with my patient was based on observation and non-verbal communication which are integral elements of every physical assessment and patient–doctor relationship.
>
> —ICM-A medical student essay, December 1990

The need for health professionals–in-training to have positive experiences that include people who have disabilities has been well documented (Gething, 1992). The important elements felt to contribute to a positive attitude formation are as follows: exposure to people with disabilities in situations in which there is a shared responsibility for the interaction between the disabled and nondisabled persons, the interaction is viewed as mutually rewarding, and there is an opportunity for the disabled person to present himself or herself as a competent and multidimensional individual (Crisp, 1987; Wright, 1983). In addition, parents of children with disabilities often complain about the way they were initially informed of their child's condition, the insensitivity of providers to their needs, and the lack of respect for parental insight and observation about their child's condition (Brynelsen, 1984; Darling, 1979; Wolraich, 1982). These experiences on the part of parents have contributed to the negative image generally held of medical providers in the health care of persons with disabilities.

Educational programs that deal with some of these concerns have been described in the literature. For the most part, these have been directed at pediatric residents (Guralnick & Richardson, 1980; Wysocki, Gururaj, Rogers, & Galey, 1987) and nursing students (Brillhart, Jay & Wyers, 1990). Medical student programs in the United States have been primarily hospital-based electives (Guild & Gunther, 1981) or limited inpatient requirements (Halstead & Halstead, 1978).

This chapter will present a description of a community-based educational experience developed at the University of Connecticut School of Medicine as part of its Introduction to Clinical Medicine (ICM) course: ICM-A, Introduction to Health and Illness from the Patient's Perspective. The assessment of the experience of thirty-two students over a four-year period, 1988–1991, will be discussed. These first-year students were matched with children who had genetic disorders that caused disability. The students visited them regularly in their homes during the first semester of medical school and participated in written and discussion exercises with faculty supervision.

This chapter describes the evolution of this unique curriculum, contains the self-described experience of the students and the children/families, and offers recommendations for generalizing this curriculum to other medical and health professions schools.

METHODS: INTRODUCTION TO CLINICAL MEDICINE—ICM-A

Introduction to Clinical Medicine is a course taught one half day each week during the first two years at the University of Connecticut School of Medicine. It has been offered continuously, with varying course formats, since the school began in 1968. It is required for all students and is designed to provide students with the basic clinical skills needed to begin their clinical clerkships in the third year. These skills form the foundation of the clinical practice of medicine and include an understanding of health and illness from the patient's perspective, effective interviewing skills, competence in taking a medical history, basic skills in physical diagnosis and assessment, and the ability to prepare effective case presentations and write-ups. There are three sections of ICM: ICM-A, Introduction to Health and Illness from the Patient's Perspective; ICM-B, Medical History and Interviewing; and ICM-C, Physical Assessment and Diagnosis.

ICM-A began in 1984. The goal was to provide entering medical students with the opportunity to have patient contact early in their medical school careers, and for them to learn the patient's perspective about health and illness before they even put on their white coats to become immersed in the technical skills of clinical medicine. The patient becomes the teacher in ICM-A, and students are encouraged to remember that patients will always be their teachers throughout their careers as doctors. The course provides an opportunity for continual patient contact outside of the hospital or health care setting. It also allows the student to examine the delivery of health care in the context of the family and its community. In addition, the course initiates modeling of peer support through small working groups of students.

Students are matched individually with patients/families who have chronic health conditions, and then the students follow these patients throughout the entire fall semester, making six to eight home visits. Patients are identified through community agencies and clinical programs at the medical school or affiliated community hospitals. Students visit patients in their homes and are expected to complete a minimum of nine contact hours during the semester. Students are encouraged to attend their patient's medical appointments and therapy sessions, and to observe the child at school, when appropriate. They then meet in small groups of eight students, two faculty, and a second-year student tutor twice a month to discuss their family experiences. In addition, they maintain a written log describing each patient visit, and complete an essay at the end of the course about their overall experience. Both the students and the patients/families evaluate the ICM-A experience. The patients have been evenly divided into pediatric and adult age groups so that discussions in the small groups cover the spectrum of age-specific issues about chronic illness. The types of chronic health conditions among the ICM-A patients are found in Table 5–1.

The course objectives generally relate to two educational areas: (1) *the health care experience of patients and families with chronic illness*; and (2) *the role development of the students as health professionals*. Students learn about community resources from the agencies and clinical programs that identified the patients, as well as from the patients and families themselves. Students also learn about the impact of chronic illness and disability on patients and their families during their visits to the patient's home and community. Cultural, economic, and social factors are explored in small group discussions and through the written student logs. Profes-

Table 5–1
Types of Chronic Conditions among ICM-A Patients

Pediatric	Adult
Diabetes	AIDS
Genetic conditions	Cardio/vascular problems
Cancer	Physical disabilities
Pulmonary problems	Elderly health problems
Sickle Cell Disease	Terminal illnesses
Other chronic illnesses	Mental illnesses
	Occupational-related disabilities
	Cancer
	Traumatic brain injury
	Other chronic illnesses

sional role development is approached through learning specific clinical skills, such as observation, listening, patient support, and obtaining a family history and the patient's social history. The student also explores issues of personal responsibility, the development of relationships with patients, limits of the doctor–patient relationship, the process of "becoming a doctor," truth-telling, and terminal illness.

The course has received positive evaluations from students, community groups, and patients. The referring clinical programs have found the student visit logs to be a valuable resource for improving patient care. Students spend considerable time with patients in their homes and often identify new and important information. The students are exposed to patients who challenge their stereotypes about disabilities, race and ethnicity, and poverty. In turn, the patients value their role as "teacher" in this course and believe that teaching students about their experiences and concerns will improve the quality of care provided by these future physicians.

In 1988, the Division of Human Genetics in the UConn Medical School Department of Pediatrics began to identify patients/families to participate in ICM-A. A total of eight patients/families from this program have subsequently participated each year, resulting in a total of thirty-two students who have worked with the program's children and their families through December 1991. Specific educational objectives were identified for the students working with these patients. They were to develop an understanding about the hereditary contribution to chronic illness; the risk

Table 5–2
ICM-A Genetics Program Participants, 1988–1991

Genetic Condition	No. Families	Genetic Condition	No. Families
PKU	4	Neurofibromatosis	2
Williams' syndrome	3	Down syndrome	7
Osteogenesis imperfecta	2	Spina bifida	1
Autism	2	Trisomy 13	1
Rubenstein-Taybi syndrome	1	Smith-Opitz-Lemli syndrome	1
Fragile X syndrome	1	Cockayne syndrome	1
Achondroplasia	1	Osteopetrosis	1
Maple Syrup Urine disease	1	Lesch-Nyhan disease	1
Turner's syndrome	1	Prader-Willi syndrome	1
		total	32

of recurrence in future pregnancies and its role in family planning; and the impact of genetic disorder–imposed disability on the extended family.

Despite the diversity of the children's health problems, the thirty-two medical students identified similar disability and long-term care issues among their patients. The two largest patient groups were children with Down syndrome and those with Phenylketonuria (PKU). Table 5–2 shows the distribution by condition among the ICM-A patients from the Division of Human Genetics program.

EVALUATION DESIGN

In order to examine the effect of this curriculum on student attitudes and knowledge about children with disabling conditions, the student logs and essays were analyzed to identify specific content areas. This was done by two different sets of reviewers. Both read the student logs and essays and classified them into several major content areas. One set of reviewers was composed of this chapter's authors. The other was an outside educator who was unaware of the ICM-A program's goals and objectives. This second analysis was conducted to control for any bias that the authors might have introduced because of their involvement in the course.

The issues identified by the authors in the student logs and essays were distributed into six major areas: (1) impact of the chronic illness on the family; (2) adapting to and coping with disability; (3) the doctor–patient relationship; (4) the importance of recognizing the individuality of the

Table 5–3
Content Areas Identified in ICM-A Student Logs and Essays, 1988–1991

Identified by Internal Review	Identified by External Review
Impact of chronic illness on family	Student's personal attitudes:
Adapting to and coping with disability	• compassion vs. pity
Doctor–patient relationship	• assessment vs. judgment
Importance of recognizing individuality of the patient	• own beliefs vs. family's beliefs
Learning clinical skills	Family dynamics
Value of patient-as-teacher experience early in medical school	Impact on family's decision making
	Impact of medical insurance issues
	Recognize patient as individual
	"Quality of life" issues
	Impact of professionals on patient and on family life
	Family's acceptance of the condition
	Beliefs and values

patient; (5) learning clinical skills; and (6) the value of the patient-as-teacher experience at the beginning of medical school. As shown in Table 5–3, there was considerable overlap between the internal and external content reviews. This suggests that there is consistency in the content areas identified by both analyses. For the purposes of further discussion, therefore, these categories will be combined.

Families also reported that they found the experience valuable. Each year, families receive a letter thanking them for their participation in the course and for their contributions to the education of the students. This letter is signed by the course director and by the dean of the medical school. A brief questionnaire is included to provide feedback on the families' experience in the course.

In an effort to assess the long-term impact of the ICM-A curriculum as but one course among many in a four-year program, a focus group discussion was held with seven of the original eight students from the 1988 ICM-A group. The purpose of this group was to determine what students remembered from ICM-A and their assessment of the value of the course to their professional development. This session lasted one hour and forty-five minutes. The discussion was taped and transcribed. Examples of issues identified by these fourth-year students will be provided later in the chapter. In general, the students felt that ICM-A had indeed affected their subsequent approach to patients with disabilities and their view of themselves as physicians.

RESULTS

Student Logs and Essays

The information in this section is arranged according to the combined content analysis areas presented in the preceding "Evaluation Design" section.

Impact of the Chronic Illness on the Family

The first content analysis area includes family dynamics and the impact of chronic illness on the family's decision making. Students often observed the effects of a chronically ill child on his or her parents, siblings, and extended family, and on social relationships outside the family. The chronic illness impacted decision making about family planning, financial hardships, and work choices related to expenses and health insurance coverage. Comments in this area were made by all thirty-two students. General family dynamics received the most attention, followed by financial problems; and thereafter, observations of the illness's impact were evenly distributed among siblings, parents, and social life.

Examples of student comments about the observed impacts follow. The age and health condition of the child/patient/teacher will be indicated first. (The patient and family initials have been changed to preserve confidentiality. In cases in which the information presented is especially sensitive, no case identification is indicated.)

Re thirteen-year-old girl with Down syndrome: I am sure A's parents would love to relax at the end of the day, watch the evening news, have a quiet dinner, put their feet up and "unwind," but they don't. Instead, when dinner is through, they share the tasks of guiding A through her homework, violin practice, nightly reading, and brushing and flossing before tucking her into bed. These don't seem like unusual parental activities at first glance, but A's parents can't simply tell her to practice her violin, read, and do her homework, because she cannot do these tasks on her own; she needs them to act as tutors every night, which clearly requires a great deal of energy and patience on their part.

Re brothers, seven and ten years old, with Maple Syrup Urine Disease: Chronically ill pediatric patients like B and C present a special problem to the health care provider. While the immediate patients are the children afflicted with the disease, the entire family feels its consequences and has to make adjustments to manage it. One striking issue that I have dealt with in this course is the enormous burden on the primary caretaker of the chronically ill pediatric patient. Since the patient is completely dependent on the caretaker for day to day living and management of the disease, there is the constant worry (especially during crisis periods), "Am I doing a good enough job in taking care of this person?"

This is exacerbated by anxiety over the possibility of death. Both the patient's and the caretaker's lives revolve around each other; so death means not only the loss of a loved one but also the end of a life's work. While the patient is still alive, however, there is anxiety about the future: Will the child do well in school or will he be able to find a job? The caretaker's job is demanding in terms of time and both physical and emotional energy, and there is danger of burnout. Moreover, there may not be time to develop other relationships which provide an important source of support.

Re ten-year-old boy with Lesch-Nyhan syndrome: The most important and obvious impression I gained from my patient was the amount of time and devotion that was required for the immediate family members in the management of D's chronic illness. Most noticeable was the effect on the patient's 17 yr. old sister who provides the majority of the care for D. She is required to give up other activities in order to care for D and therefore has suffered in terms of her own social development. In addition, the mother and father have had to make changes in their lifestyles, most noticeably being their work schedules: the father took on a second part-time job to help with expenses and the mother was required to shift to 2nd shift in order to be available for D when the others aren't around. The end result has been a severe strain on the family's quality time and also has led to a possible overdependence on the sister. I truly wonder what the future will hold for the family when the sister has to make decisions concerning her future educational and marriage plans.

Decision making about having other children was also observed in the families.

Re seven-year-old girl with osteogenesis imperfecta (OI): They decided to have the second child after weighing the chances of another OI child. Mr. A had to convince Mrs. A not to have a child right away, because as she admits, there was a time she wanted to fill a gap, or prove something. Before their second child was born, she had a miscarriage first. So she was "carrying a lot of baggage" by the time the second child was born. . . . Mr. A mentioned that it took her a while to feel that "maternal feeling" towards the second child, because she's built up walls to protect herself, in case of what might happen. The third child was unplanned but very healthy. Mrs. A just had her tubes tied a few weeks ago, "to avoid any more possibility."

The effect on marital relationships was noted in another family.

For a long time Mr. B blamed her for having the kids, and he was embarrassed to take her out. He was frustrated, drank, was verbally abusive, and blamed her for his drinking problem. His family was cold toward Mrs. B.

The differing needs of family members was also identified.

Re ten-month-old boy with achondroplasia: I also was exposed to different needs in parents at the time of learning about a child's disease. Mrs. C flat out said she could care less about hearing the chances of her baby having a baby with the same disease. In fact, she thought it was inappropriate to hear this information just as she learned about her son having achondroplasia. Meanwhile, Mr. C was taking notes about these details. Both parents had very different needs at the time of E's birth. I imagine that is difficult for a physician to balance these needs when consulting both parents.

Another related area was the isolation that parents experience because they are reluctant to leave their disabled child with anyone else. Some students actually provided some respite care to the parents after they got to know the child and family well, thus demonstrating a sense of responsibility to assist with problems identified.

The interplay of family dynamics and patient care was another area that was discussed. In families where the parents' relationships were strained, or other stress and coping problems existed within the family, students observed the effect this had on the family's ability to care for the child and follow therapeutic regimens.

Adapting to and Coping with Disability

The area of adapting and coping includes the family's acceptance of the condition, their beliefs and values, and "quality of life" issues. All students reported discussing the family's adaptation to the child's diagnosis, and most identified the sense of loss that parents feel at not having a "normal" child. These issues required a clarification of values for many students because the coping style and strategies employed by their patient/teacher families sometimes conflicted with their own religious, moral, or scientific beliefs.

Mourning the loss of the expected "normal" child was identified by several students and families, along with "stages" of family adjustment.

Re ten-month-old boy with achondroplasia: As expected, one would imagine disappointment at the loss of the "perfect child." For E's parents this was the case. One image they shared with me, was the notion of "burying the perfect baby" when they learned of E's disease. I found myself torn by what appeared to me a harsh way of viewing the situation. I realized then that I had to withhold my own opinions and feelings in order to be an objective supportive listener. Overall, I felt that my listening skills had not changed, but my role as a listener did change. Now I was imagining what it would be like to listen as a "doctor."

Quality of life was another issue the students found a need to address.

Re two-year-old girl with Rubenstein-Taybi syndrome: I think that the "normal" baby is so pervasive in the books, advertising and general media of our society that we are saturated by these images and therefore have very narrow and high expectations. I thought that getting to know H would enlighten me on the life of a retarded child, but I have found that it revealed the disabilities I have inherited from my society. H's physical and mental development were considerably delayed yet she is a tremendous person. I found myself asking, what defines the quality of a person's life? The constant push for "success" in our society has resulted in success being representative of quality. . . . In some ways H may be lucky, for there is no "normal" for her development.

Re three-year-old girl with Type II osteogenesis imperfecta in an adoptive group home: When I first met J two months ago, I was very upset about the physical consequences of osteogenesis imperfecta. I remember asking, "What kind of life for a little girl is this?" Now, when I play with her, I no longer see just her crooked bones. I still feel sad that she'll never be able to walk or run across the room or even sit up on her own, but I don't dwell on that anymore. Instead, I get excited when she says a new word, recognized Big Bird on the tv, wiggles her toes or waves her arms and legs to the beat of the music she hears. I think that I've gotten to know J, not just as a baby with OI, but as a little person. J is a wonderfully happy baby. . . . A major reason for my change of attitude regarding OI and J is probably that I've stopped comparing her development to that of a "normal" child. I realize now that J does have a life. She will grow and develop, but at her own pace and in her own special way.

One example of different belief systems dealt with religious beliefs.

Re five-month-old twin sisters with PKU: Much of the support for the family comes from their religious beliefs and their church. Mrs. E feels that God gave K and L PKU for a reason, and, while they may never know what that reason is, it is comforting to feel that there is a plan. I must say that I was personally somewhat distressed at this attitude, until I began to get to know the family better. It seemed to me too simplistic a view by which to live life. I have never been able to accept the idea that God makes bad things to happen to good people for a reason. It was, therefore, very difficult for me to understand Mrs. E's point of view. As time went on, however, I began to see that this belief made dealing with the problems of PKU very straightforward.

Understanding parent views about causation was also identified by students.

Re five-year-old girl with Williams' syndrome: Mrs. F when asked about her daughter's condition alluded to possible causes such as her British heritage and the fact that M's pregnancy was long after her previous pregnancy (12 years). Although the cause of Williams' syndrome remains a mystery and is probably not linked to either of Mrs. F's explanations, I believe that it is important to listen to a patient and attempt to understand his/her views.

The importance of positive parent attitudes was also identified.

Re three-year-old child with Down syndrome: In general, this experience has shown me how other people deal with illness, and how important a positive attitude is. From my interaction with my patient and her family, I believe that I could deal with having a handicapped child myself.

Parent belief systems were clearly identified as important areas. One example was a child with slow weight gain for whom the doctor recommended surgical implantation of a feeding tube (gastrostomy).

N's father agrees with the doctor. Mrs. G, on the other hand, does not want the procedure done. She feels the doctors are playing God. She feels that God has a purpose for N and that she does not want to impede that. I don't think Mrs. G has been told all the benefits that N may derive from the procedure. She feels it is going to be more difficult in caring for N. She feels that Mr. G agreed to it only because he would not have to deal with the new procedure.

Later, after the operation was scheduled, the student discovered that

Mrs. G was indecisive about the operation because she thought the tubes would be placed through the belly button. She doesn't think anyone should be fooling around with the belly button. When she found out tubes would be placed in N's side, she agreed.

Doctor–Patient Relationship

The doctor–patient relationship issues identified by the students included the role of physicians in diagnosing, informing, treating, and responding to parent concerns, as well as the role of health professionals in patient and family life. Family frustration about the way they were informed of the child's condition, and about the way doctors responded to their concerns over illness and treatment, was a common theme in the logs and essays of many of the students.

One student noted that the physician has a responsibility to provide information to parents about family support groups.

Re three-year-old girl with Down syndrome: The physician is usually the first person who diagnoses an illness and is therefore the first person who the patient is in contact with. I believe that it is very important for the physician to have a knowledge of, or easy access to, information about support systems in the immediate area.

Individuality of the Patient

Another issue/content area dealt with the existence of student-held stereotypes, the breakdown of these stereotypes, and the need to learn about the individual capacities of patients.

Re three-year-old girl with Type II osteogenesis imperfecta, in an adoptive group home: One of the biggest things I learned was that each one of these children, no matter how severely disabled, is a special and unique individual with their own individual developmental milestones, achievement, and triumphs to celebrate. . . . Although I have personal experience with chronic illness in my own family, this experience showed me how individual each experience is, and how important it is not to assume the chronically ill, and their families, have the same problems and circumstances.

Re fifteen-month-old boy with Prader-Willi syndrome: I have come to see G as a playful, loving little boy, and not simply a "child with Prader-Willi." I think this will be an important lesson to remember when dealing with all patients.

Re ten-month-old boy with achondroplasia: I was very pleasantly surprised to see how alert and aware E was of his surroundings. It really made me think positively about E as an individual, rather than, "poor E with the genetic disease." It gave me much to reflect upon afterwards in regards to my own perception of genetic disorders and the "diseased state" in general.

A few students had personal experience with some of the behavioral problems of their patients; they seemed to take it in stride as a part of their education.

Re ten-year-old boy with Lesch-Nyhan syndrome: During this visit, I had the best contact with the patient himself, as most visits have been predominantly spent talking with his family. The patient frequently hits others around him, as this is a regular behavioral symptom of his condition and I was struck by D for the first time when I was initially speaking to him. While I was talking to him about his school, he just reached over and slapped me in the face. I was taken by surprise and really didn't know how to react, but I did soon recall that this was something that frequently happened with the patient and that he really had no control over his actions.

Learning Clinical Skills

The students wrote about issues of professional responsibility, the development of listening skills, the importance of observation, "becoming a doctor," participation of the patient in treatment decisions, the need to withhold value judgments, and their own discovery of the difference between compassion and pity. Many of these issues have been illustrated in the preceding excerpts; there were many other such instances in the students' writing, as, for example, the following:

Re ten-month-old boy with achondroplasia: I thought I would "feel sorry" for E and his parents. So much to my surprise, it was not that way. I was amazed at how happy I felt for them, mainly because of their love for their child. I felt lucky to be introduced to such a positive situation early on. Genetic disorders often have depressive connotations, and E and his family really helped me learn that a genetic disease or a chronic illness does not have to be a depressing ordeal.

The same student commented in her essay,

For myself I hope I can impart the will, strength, and patience that this family has shown me, to others coping with similar illnesses.

One student who was working with a two-year-old child with osteopetrosis in the terminal stages of her illness made some particularly poignant observations.

Above all, no one can really see what this family experiences. I think I see a window into their life: their daily routines, their minor setbacks offset by victories. One of their most fervent desires is to make me understand that I cannot feel their painful experience, but that I should recognize and acknowledge it and incorporate this into my fiber as a professional. Another lesson: chronic illness does not stop when the patient leaves the office; it is a way of life. . . . I wonder if some physicians do feel helpless (as I do when I listen to the pained words of my patient's family) and try to move further away instead of closer. . . . It is very difficult to witness Q's conditions deteriorate. Somehow, however, I am becoming more comfortable as I lend *my* support to Q and her family. There is some sort of lesson here, although I don't think I fully understand it yet. It is something about the value of having a relationship that is close enough to be painful.

Value of Patient-as-Teacher Experience

Many students commented on the value of ICM-A early in their medical school training. It was often viewed as "the light at the end of the tunnel" and reminded them of why they were interested in medicine as a career.

Re nine-year-old boy with Down syndrome: Before I began my visits with P's family, I was uncomfortable around handicapped children. After my experience with this family, I have conquered most of my fears and feel I would like to work with the mentally handicapped in the future.

Re three-year-old girl with osteogenesis imperfecta: ICM-A has truly been the best part of medical school so far. My decision to become a medical doctor was based largely on the fact that I enjoy working with people—especially children. The opportunity which ICM-A gave me to have contact with patients outside of the medical school helped keep that end in sight. I looked forward to visiting my patient and her family every week. Not only was it a needed break from the books, but it also helped put things into proper perspective. After spending most of every day in lecture or alone studying, it is very easy to forget that behind all these abnormal cells and diseases we are learning about are real people.

This type of experience early in a medical student's career can create a lasting impression about the importance of listening to and providing support for families of children with special needs.

Re seventeen-month-old boy with Down syndrome: If I am able to remember a small portion of all that I have heard and seen in my ICM-A experience, I feel I and the medical profession will benefit greatly. The ICM-A program allowed me to remain focused on my goal of a health care provider as I sank deeper in the endless, seemingly useless facts of CMB [basic science course]. ICM-A was the one time each week when I was able to sit back, listen, and think critically not for the sake of a test but for the sake of another human being.

Patient/Family Response to ICM-A

At the end of the course, questionnaires that asked for feedback were included with the thank-you letters sent to participating families. It was not possible to link family evaluations with matched students until the 1989 schoolyear. Thus, families identified by the Division of Human Genetics program could only be linked for three of the four groups of ICM-A students, or twenty-four of the thirty-two students. There was a 75 percent response rate from the twenty-four eligible families. This compares favorably with the response rate for the entire class for this same period. The questions sent to the families are presented in Table 5–4; this table also includes results for the closed-ended questions.

The majority of families rated the experience as excellent, the highest rating. They were very satisfied (100%) with the frequency of the visits, which was either every week or every other week for most (72%) of the families. They also found the length of the visit to be satisfactory (100% of those responding); the average length of a visit was one and a half hours. The frequency and length of the visits were established by mutual

Table 5–4
ICM-A Genetics Program Parent Responses, 1989–1991: Questionnaire, and Closed-ended Results

1. How would you rate the experience in general?
   78% excellent   22% good   ok   bad
2. How often did the student visit?
   44% 1/wk   28% alt/wk   28% other
3. Was this amount of visiting
   too often   not enough   100% just right
4. Did you fully understand, in the beginning, that these visits would stop at the end of the fall semester?
   94% yes   6%* no response
5. How long did each visit usually last?
   1½ hours
6. Was this amount of time
   too long   not enough   94% just right
   6%* no response
7. Did you receive enough information about the program before you started?
   67% yes   28% no   6%* not sure
8. Did you understand your role as "teacher" in this program?
   78% yes   17% no   6%* not sure
9. Do you have any recommendations for next year?
10. Do you have any general comments about the program or the student?
11. Would you be interested in participating in this program next year (with a new student)?
    78% yes   6%* no   17% maybe

*$N = 1$

agreement between the medical student and the family, so this level of satisfaction is not surprising.

In terms of how well the families understood the program *before* it commenced, all of those responding indicated they understood the visits would stop at the end of the semester, 78 percent understood their role as a teacher in the program, and 67 percent felt they had received enough information before the course began.

The response to the open-ended questions was also positive. Families were asked for general comments about the program or the student. Examples of these responses include the following:

> [Student] is a very dedicated young lady.
>
> [Student] was a pleasure and will make a fine doctor.
>
> [Student] is a nice young man and the kids liked him very much.
>
> I think it's wonderful, what you're doing for the students. I'm sure it'll make them more compassionate doctors.

Favorable comments about the students were found in 75 percent of the responses.

Favorable general statements about the program were found in 58 percent of the responses. There were no absolutely negative responses. Specific suggestions for improving the program included these: providing families with more information about the goals of the program ($n = 3$); giving students more information about the child's health condition ($n = 1$) or more guidance on what questions to ask ($n = 1$); and having students repeat this experience as a resident ($n = 1$).

A few families provided more detailed responses about the meaning of the experience, as in the following:

> We enjoyed having [student] in our home. We hope we helped him understand patients and their families better. Hope the program stays for many years—if even one student gets a better understanding, your program will have been a success.
>
> We learned as much about aspiring physicians as I'm sure [student] learned from us—it was equally beneficial.
>
> [Student] was a terrific young woman. Her enthusiasm was contagious. We had a great time working with her. While we were initially unsure about what this program would entail, we quickly got involved. We sincerely hope that she learned as much from us as we did from her. This is an excellent program which has given us a chance to see the reasons behind the questions.

Although we generally preferred not to use the same families in subsequent years, families were asked whether they would be interested in participating again the following year. This represented another measure of satisfaction with the course, although the response was also likely to be influenced by other issues. The majority (78%) of families responded that they would be interested in participating again. In addition, three families indicated that they might be interested, depending on how the child was doing. Only one family indicated that they would not be interested; limited availability of time, and the health condition of the caretaker, were given as reasons. One of the uncertain families gave a lengthy and rich response.

> We'll have to see about next fall's class. The one thing we didn't realize up front was how much time it really involves. Our young, busy family finds it tough to set aside one evening/week for three+ months, though fortunately [student] was an *absolute* pleasure!
>
> Reliving the past was emotionally draining—much to our surprise! We thought we had dealt with many of "those feelings" and buried them years ago. Both [husband] and I found that painful, though knowing it was going to help [student] made it worthwhile. Perhaps a year off *is* in order. The program gave us more than we gave to it. We developed a wonderful relationship, and will continue to be interested in [student]'s successes and progress.

Continuing Impact on Students

In 1991, the fourth-year students who had been enrolled in ICM-A in 1988 were invited to participate in a focus group about whether there was a continuing effect of the ICM-A course on their subsequent medical school experiences. Seven of the eight students were able to attend; the eighth was in California and was interviewed by telephone. The students were sent an invitation indicating that two major areas would be explored in the discussion:

1. Has the ICM-A experience affected your perception of and work with children and adults with disabilities?
2. Did this experience influence in any way your choice of career?

The students were also asked to bring up other issues they felt were important to the discussion. They were each mailed a copy of their own 1988 ICM-A essay to review prior to the discussion. The invitation indicated that the session would be tape-recorded.

The discussion was held in the evening at the home of one of the authors and was followed by dinner. The discussion lasted one and a half hours and began with each student describing his or her ICM-A patient and family to the group. This evolved into a discussion of the role of ICM-A in the context of the many learning experiences and influences the students had experienced since the first year.

Most of the students felt there had definitely been an influence, because ICM-A had provided them their "first patient" experience. This is illustrated by the following response:

R was the first patient I ever had and I got to meet him without any IVs and tubes in him, in the context of his own home, wearing normal clothing, in a supportive environment with his relatives all around. And I didn't really realize it, but now that I think back—when I look at patients in the hospital, I always try to think about what they look like on the street. I always imagine them wearing regular clothes, and I try to separate them from their patient role. I never really made a connection until I started to think about it, but I think it's because the first patient I ever knew was not in the hospital. And it was a very good experience.

It seemed the first patient experience was a less powerful influence for those students who had previous clinical experiences and/or interactions with children with disabilities. One student's own mother taught special education, and so the student felt this was not such a "new" experience for her. Another had worked as an emergency medical technician for six years prior to medical school. He had also known a child and family with a rare genetic condition and had worked with them over a period of time. However, most students had no prior exposure to disability or mental retardation; ICM-A gave them a chance to explore their values and prejudices, as well as learn about their patient and family's views.

One of the themes that developed during the discussion was that ICM-A was a "shock." This comment was generated by the significant influence the child and family contact had as a first patient experience. Some students felt shocked, but some felt that the shock was not great compared to the intensity of other medical school experiences. Other students felt it was simply part of a four-year continuum of experiences.

Many of the issues originally noted in the student logs and essay reemerged in the focus group, especially those of changing stereotypes, quality of life, observing family dynamics, and the impact of chronic illness on the family. There was a general consensus that seeing patients in their homes, and getting to know the family, permitted an emphasis on the patient as a "whole person," not just as a disease. Some of the previous excerpts illustrated this point; but one example, in particular, from the focus group discussion may add further insight to this issue.

This experience dealing with young children in a family situation—[with a] focus on the dynamics, how it affects and fits into the whole family—makes you think later on when you look at adults. It's almost comparable in a funny way to an elderly parent who's dependent and being taken care of at home. I haven't dealt with that many young children who are as impaired as H; but certainly when I saw patients with Alzheimer's or other dementias being cared for at home or in nursing homes, it made me think of how they interact with their families. I don't know if that stems directly from this experience, but it definitely is related.

The need to reinforce the educational objectives of ICM-A throughout medical school was identified during the discussion. The students expressed concern that the demands of the third-year clerkships—especially the intensive inpatient experiences, combined with the realities of the limitations imposed by health care financing—made it difficult for them to maintain the humanistic orientation they learned in ICM-A. The group unanimously agreed that all students should review their ICM-A essays in the fourth year. They felt this would serve several purposes: to give students perspective on how they've grown personally and professionally; to provide insight into the humanistic principles they want to maintain in patient care; and to remind them of the importance of patient and family perspectives. The group also felt it would be valuable for all students to participate in a fourth-year focus group as a reinforcement technique.

It is clear from the results of the focus group discussion that the students feel their experiences in ICM-A had a positive influence on their perceptions of children and adults with disabilities. However, the experience apparently had not influenced their choice of career. Most of the students had already had an idea of the specialty they were interested in when they first began medical school. The residency selections of the students from the ICM-A group of 1988 were surgery (3), pediatrics (2), obstetrics and gynecology (1), emergency medicine (1), and anesthesia (1). Those students who chose pediatrics felt that ICM-A had helped convince them this was the right choice, and felt that they would continue to apply what they had learned. The other students also felt that ICM-A would continue to be of value, even though they would not be working directly with children.

DISCUSSION

The traditional medical school curriculum has been a fact-based lockstep series of courses that emphasizes memorization and test-taking over affective experiences. This chapter has described an attempt to develop and implement, early in the curriculum, a course that teaches medical students about the impact of chronic or disabling disorders on patients and families. The course was developed by the senior author, who had previously taught students in the hospital-based ICM course. She had found that students had a great deal of difficulty asking personal questions—primarily those related to the social history part of the data base. Students felt that asking questions about a patient's age, level of education, marital status, living arrangements, financial situation, and employment was intrusive and not necessarily related to the patient's *medical* condition. Questions about chief complaint, past medical history, and review of systems were viewed as relevant and appropriate. ICM-A was therefore designed to place students in a patient's home environment so that they could learn the relevance of "social areas" to the patient's health and illness. The course was also structured so that students would view patients as their teachers throughout their clinical careers. This point is made in the syllabus and course orientation: Patients *always* know the most about their experience of illness. Listening and observation are identified as two critical professional skills and, for first-year students, the main skills they have available to practice and refine.

Meeting the ICM-A's Overall Course Objectives

The overall educational goals of ICM-A were developed for the entire class, and they can be listed as follows:

- Development of professional skills in the areas of observation and listening
- Ability to establish and complete a one-to-one relationship with a patient and/or family
- Ability to conceptualize the meaning and impact of chronic illness on patient, environment, and lifestyle
- Ability to exchange constructive verbal feedback with peers
- Ability to establish a group relationship and make significant contributions
- Development of awareness of student's own feelings, attitudes, and judgments about patients, illness, and the health care system
- Ability to take and record a family and social history in a standard format

These objectives reflect the developmental level of the first-year students, who are eager to pursue "real" patient experiences at the same time that they are immersed in the basic science curriculum.

The results of various evaluations—including the student logs and essays, the family questionnaires, the student focus group, and the two content analyses of the written materials—indicate that all the objectives were indeed fulfilled by the students we studied. Whether the course experience has the desired lasting impact on the students is more difficult to determine. This is an issue that confronts all educational endeavors in the medical school curriculum because of its enormous scope, breadth, and intensity. A more rigorous research design that permitted a greater number of students to be followed throughout the four-year medical school experience, and beyond, would be necessary to determine the true "impact" of the ICM-A course.

The ICM-A Genetics Course Objectives

The addition of the genetics objectives were expected to enhance the ICM-A objectives by further illuminating other family dynamics, such as the issue of reproductive risk on family planning, or the familial contribution of heredity to a genetic disorder. These objectives were accomplished, as evidenced by the information in the logs and essays. Students did learn about families' reproductive decision-making and understanding of risk and causation. They also found out that timing was important in terms of when parents wanted to know this information, and that these preferences varied within families as well as among families. Because all of the students obtained a family history that included a genogram, these students were able to identify the extent and impact of genetic disorders in the extended family. In addition to the eight students each year who were matched with children from the Division of Human Genetics, there were eight other students in their group discussions, resulting in sixty-four students in this four-year period who learned about the genetic objectives. Future plans for the course include making sure that every group has a student matched with a child with special needs. This would give all the ICM-A students the opportunity to explore the issues faced by these children and their families.

Course Structure

The authors found that obtaining and retaining families for the ICM-A experience was not difficult. Individual treating physicians and community programs indicated that most families were pleased to be asked, valued their role as teachers of medical students, and provided valuable feedback to the faculty and students.

Overall, the ICM-A students were matched to clinical programs based on their preference to work with children or adults and their clinical areas of interest—such as neurological, genetic, and so forth—when these are indicated. The matching of students with specific patents/families in the Division of Human Genetics was accomplished via a meeting of the group of eight students with the second author, who would describe the patients' individual conditions and then answer questions about the families. The students then self-selected their families based on personal interests and proximity to the student's residence, since the visits to the families were usually in the evening. As described, the number of visits ranged from six to nine, depending on mutually agreed conditions between the student and the family.

A critical component of the ICM-A course is the timely submission of students' logs to their faculty preceptors. The syllabus indicates that logs must be submitted within forty-eight hours of a student's visit. Unfortunately, logs were often not submitted within this time period. This delay resulted from the demands of the basic science course work, and the fact that the information could be conveyed orally during the group sessions every other week. Without the written logs, the faculty had a difficult job providing timely feedback to students, and were limited in their ability to assist students with problems encountered in relationships with the families. However, there were many opportunities for both group and individual student problem-solving—a process that helped to reinforce the ICM-A objectives as the semester progressed.

One of the most difficult processes for the students was in ending the relationship and separating from the experience. Since this was a first patient experience, many students became very involved and enmeshed with the family, making it difficult for them to say goodbye. However, while this was painful for some students, we believe that it is important for them to learn to acknowledge transition points in their relationships with patients. There is no hard-and-fast rule that students shouldn't see their ICM-A patients again, but they must let the families know that their level of involvement will decrease because of their changing educational responsibilities. Most of the families understood that the course would end, and they recognized the importance of students' needing to learn strategies for ending doctor–patient relationships. Alternatively, we sometimes found it necessary to push some students forward in order to engage them more effectively with the family. These students were hesitant about dealing with affective and psychosocial issues. But such situations, as well as ending the course relationship, provided opportunities for the students—during the group discussions—to support each other, discuss different approaches, and reflect on their own feelings.

As noted at the end of the "Results" section, there is very little time or opportunity in years two, three, and four to reassemble medical students in order to explore ICM-A issues. The fourth-year-student focus group voiced a collective concern that the affective and humanistic issues surrounding or emerging from patient care are frequently overlooked, or at least are not dealt with in a timely or effective manner. Because UConn medical school is undergoing a major curriculum revision, there is now an opportunity to develop a continuing ICM curriculum in order to keep the small groups intact during the third and fourth years. This would reinforce the ICM-A experience and support students as they face other challenging patient-care situations during their clinical training.

CONCLUSIONS

The ICM-A course described in this chapter has been successful in meeting its objectives of teaching medical students about child and parent views of chronic and disabling conditions. Its success in dealing with stereotypes about disability and in providing positive images for health professionals is derived from meeting several conditions cited at the beginning of the chapter. *There is shared responsibility for the interaction between the disabled and nondisabled person.* This occurs through the invitation to children and families to participate, through the negotiation of meeting times, duration, and frequency between the student and the family, and through the setting of specific goals for the interaction between the student and the family. *The interaction is viewed as mutually rewarding.* The families participate in the course because they want to help future doctors become more sensitive to child and family concerns; the students view the children and families as their teachers about the experience of health and illness. *There is an opportunity for the disabled person to present himself or herself as a competent and multidimensional individual.* Visiting children and families at home and in the community provides the students with the broadest possible view of children with disabilities and the role of families in their care. These three areas are well documented in the ICM-A student logs and essays.

This course represents a partnership between the medical school and patients/families in order to provide better educational experiences about patients' needs and their perceptions of chronic and disabling conditions. It is a model that should be adopted by other medical schools, and that could be adapted for the education of other health professionals.

ACKNOWLEDGMENTS

The authors wish to express their thanks to Arlene Greenstein for her contributions to the content analysis of the student logs and essays. They also wish to thank Patricia Giomblanco and Charlotte Politis for their many contributions to the ICM-A course.

REFERENCES

Brillhart, B. A., Jay, H., & Wyers, M. E. (1990). Attitudes toward people with disabilities. *Rehabilitation Nursing* 15:80–85.

Brynelsen, D., ed. (1984). *Working together: A handbook for parents and professionals.* Toronto: National Institute on Mental Retardation.

Crisp, R. (1987). Helping relationships: Key issues. *Australian Disabilities Review* 4:56–59.

Darling, R. B. (1979). *Families against society: A study of reactions to children with birth defects.* Beverly Hills, CA: Sage.

Gething, L. (1992). Judgements by health professionals of personal characteristics of people with a visible physical disability. *Social Science and Medicine* 34:809–815.

Guild, S., & Gunter, M. S. (1981). Patient perspectives program: A humanistic educational experience for medical students. *Archives of Physical Medicine Rehabilitation* 62:461–466.

Guralnick, M. J., & Richardson, H. B., Jr. (1980). *Pediatric education and the needs of exceptional children.* Baltimore: University Park Press.

Halstead, L. S., & Halstead, M. (1978). Chronic illness and humanism: Rehabilitation as a model for teaching humanistic and scientific health care. *Archives of Physical Medicine Rehabilitation* 59:53–57.

Wolraich, M. L. (1982). Communication between physicians and parents of handicapped children. *Exceptional Children* 48:324–329.

Wright, B. A. (1983). *Physical disability: A psychosocial approach.* New York: Harper & Row.

Wysocki, T., Gururaj, V., Rogers, M. A., & Galey, G. (1987). Training pediatric residents in early intervention with handicapped children. *Journal of Medical Education* 62:47–52.

6

Parents as Educators of Medical Students

Nancy J. DiVenere

The Medical Education Project began as a collaborative venture, a partnership between the University of Vermont College of Medicine and the organization Parent to Parent of Vermont.[1] It began as an opportunity for medical students to learn the art of practicing medicine from families and individuals themselves.

In 1984, an apparent lack of appropriate treatment of persons with disabilities in the emergency room of a Vermont hospital prompted a response from advocates as well as hospital staff and administrators. A network of parents whose children have a chronic illness or disability grew to become Parent to Parent, which has provided an ideal forum for discussion and eventual resolution of the question of how to influence the attitudes of care providers toward persons with disabilities.

Two physicians serving on the board of directors of Parent to Parent of Vermont—Donald Swartz and David Stifler—suggested introducing a series of lectures for third-year medical students that would be punctuated by a student visit to the home of a family or individual experiencing chronic illness or disability. This model of physician education—now the Medical Education Project—has proven to be an invaluable experience for medical students, as shown by the following statements:

> In the three hours I was with the family I heard how physicians should listen more. I also learned that this family needed to have relationships and feel comfortable with their child's physician.

The pediatrician's attitude made a difference. It has been since they [the family] were told. The pediatrician came into the room, sat down with them, and talked to them. He [the father] said if the pediatrician had not had that attitude the information would have been devastating.

It is a very valuable time for students. Not only do students learn something they could never learn in school; it also allows the parents to feel they are making an impact on future doctors.

The Medical Education Project is designed to encourage students to recognize and evaluate their own personal biases and beliefs toward chronic illness and disability; enhance their knowledge and understanding of family-centered care; and acknowledge and integrate the experience and insight of persons with a chronic illness or disability and their families. On the students' end, this agenda is accomplished through three required sessions: (1) introductory student lecture and discussion; (2) the home visit; and (3) follow-up student lecture and discussion. The fourth—and primary—component of the Medical Education Project, however, is that of family recruitment and orientation.

FAMILY RECRUITMENT AND ORIENTATION

Parent to Parent of Vermont is a statewide nonprofit organization offering families a variety of emotional supports, including one-to-one peer support, information and access to community, state, and national resources, and an opportunity for families to use their experiences to enhance the education of future health-care providers and educators. More than eight hundred families are involved in this network. Forty percent of the families reside in Chittenden County, home to the office of Parent to Parent of Vermont, the University of Vermont College of Medicine, and the Medical Center Hospital of Vermont.

One-to-one peer support—the opportunity to talk with other parents who have shared a similar experience—is the primary reason families contact Parent to Parent. Families are in touch with Parent to Parent daily. Family concerns range from health care financing to finding quality childcare. For many families who call Parent to Parent, the need for information about their child's diagnosis is paramount. How will they tell family and friends? How do other families manage multiple demands and expectations? Are necessary services and supports available in their community? And how are they accessed? Each call from a family presents a different set of concerns; each one summons a different response. All families in the network are singularly prepared for their role as "community faculty."

Of the families involved in Parent to Parent, forty-two presently participate in the Medical Education Project. Recruitment is ongoing. Letters from Parent to Parent and physicians involved in the project are sent to potential participants semiannually. The letter includes anecdotal comments from participating students and families. Comments from students following a home visit provide additional incentives to families already confident that they have a message to share with future providers of care. Many families self-select to participate, others are encouraged by health care providers and educators who believe that a particular family's experience would offer exceptional insight.

The forty-two families represent a wide range of chronic illnesses and disabilities. During the two-hour orientation held four times a year, families have an opportunity to hear about the evolution and intent of the project, to talk with families presently involved, and to begin considering the message they would like to get across to medical students during the home visit. Families are asked to identify three points they would like to make during the visit with students and to consider how best to convey that message.

What has been so exceptional about this project is the collaboration, commitment, and support of Dr. Carol Phillips, chair of the Department of Pediatrics at the University of Vermont College of Medicine. The endorsement she wrote has been highly instrumental to the recruitment of families; it reads as follows:

> I can easily tell which students have had the experience with one of your [Parent to Parent] families by their eagerness to discuss plans with parents and have a joint decision-making process. Students eagerly tell me of their experiences with "their" family and how much it influenced them.

Student comments from past home visits are shared with families during the project's orientation sessions. These statements provide reassurance that the family perspective can make a difference.

> Until you have heard the story and seen some of the daily activities of a family with a child with special needs, you can't understand the effect on their lives. Visits to the home are rare in medical school but essential for the well-rounded perspective.

> I think that it is very difficult to have a good idea of what having a child with a disability is like without seeing the child in his room and interacting with the family. It was very interesting to get the child's viewpoint on how he felt about himself and what he felt others thought about it [his disability]. I really enjoyed meeting with the child and was very impressed with how active he was.

INTRODUCTORY STUDENT LECTURE AND DISCUSSION

The introductory student lecture and discussion take place during the first week of clinical rotation in pediatrics—a time when students are acquiring technical skills and developing their own personal styles of interaction. Students come to the lecture with notebooks and pens, prepared for a typical medical school lecture. They quickly learn that this lecture is out of the ordinary, however.

Right away, students are asked to respond to the following question: As a parent, which of the following four diagnoses would you find easiest to cope with, and which the most difficult, and why? These are the four choices: cystic fibrosis; Down syndrome; meningomyelocele; or disfiguring third-degree burns. "Votes" are initially tallied anonymously, the results charted and shared. Typically, the results show an even distribution of choices. Each student then discusses how he or she voted, and why. It becomes clear during this discussion that everyone has biases, many of which are not necessarily based on facts about the illness or disability. Students observe that they do not need to know anything to have an opinion!

This discussion helps medical students understand that they are bringing to the practice of medicine their own unique styles of interaction, their own values, their own set of biases and beliefs. And, as becomes evident during the session, students who have had a personal experience or relationship with an individual or family with a chronic illness or disability bring to the discussion a perception and understanding far different from those of their peers. Ultimately, the attitudes of all the students will be further enlightened or strengthened by the home visit experience.

A little anecdote should serve to illustrate the significance of this introductory lecture: When asked which diagnosis would be the most difficult—and which the easiest—to cope with, one student replied, "I would find cystic fibrosis the easiest because with cystic fibrosis there is a treatment." The next student said, "I would find cystic fibrosis the hardest because of recurrent hospitalizations and the difficulty of seeing your child constantly hospitalized."

Dr. Swartz recalls for the students what he himself had learned from a family: that treatment can be a constant reminder, a daily reminder, that the child may not survive adolescence. For such a family, a sudden need for hospitalization may be welcome relief from a demanding, heartrending therapy. The choices articulated by the students—as they have begun to realize—reflect personal biases that may influence their professional decision making in such a situation.

Dr. Stifler often reminds students that "we can know the wrong things or have outdated information. The information the parents get has been filtered through your understanding of the problem and this can color how the family hears information."

The observations of Drs. Swartz and Stifler are essential to the success of this introductory session. Their personal reflections and responses guide students to appreciate more fully this unique learning experience.

THE HOME VISIT

Parent to Parent of Vermont believes that a relationship between family/individual and physician that encourages honest and open communication, embraces mutual respect, acknowledges expectations, and demonstrates care and concern is essential to successful outcomes for children and their families. The home is the setting for a unique opportunity to rehearse this necessary relationship and to acquire essential skills. Families—as "community faculty"—open their homes and share their experiences. The content of this teaching session is the family's experience.

Families are asked to host one or two medical students per year and are encouraged to have medical students visit at a time most consistent with their message and most convenient for their family. Many families invite students for dinner, or to spend an afternoon. The length of the visit is determined by the family and has never been an issue of concern for either students or families. Students are given no information about the child or family prior to their home visit. This is an uncomfortable situation for many students—a role reversal of sorts. Students are no longer in the hospital, clinic, or office setting; they are on unfamiliar turf. The family is in control.

Prior to the home visit, families are asked to write down the message they would want to get across to the medical student. The following is how one family responded:

What are the major points that you want to get across during the visit?

a. Our daughter is a beautiful, fun little girl who is a joy to be around.
b. Our daughter is not that different from other kids—and that we are a normal family.

c. We are just like any other parents raising their children.

Another family identified the following points:

a. Doctors should be open and honest with their patients. If they don't know, say they don't know. Don't skirt the issue.
b. Our daughter is a person first and not a diagnosis and deserves to be treated with respect.

And another family:

a. Physicians need to be sensitive to family concerns and needs. Listen and respect them. They know their child and family best.
b. Parent's emotional adjustment is a journey. It doesn't end when a diagnosis is given.

Asking parents to write these messages beforehand assists them in guiding and directing the home visit.

FOLLOW-UP STUDENT LECTURE AND DISCUSSION

At the follow-up lecture and discussion, facilitated by Drs. Swartz and Stifler, students are asked to relate their home visit experiences. Each story reaffirms the central role the family plays in the life of the child patient. Each visit offers yet another perspective—another glimpse at the reality of health care and another hint about the qualities of a successful relationship between parents and physicians. The messages brought to the table by the students provide fruitful dialogue for this follow-up session.

One student reported it was the family's positive attitude toward their daughter that had made a difference in her development—in contrast to the attitude that had met them at the hospital following their daughter's delivery.

> She [the mother] said that, when she was about to leave the hospital, her physician asked if she had gotten all the information that new families get and she said no. She began to think that she had been ignored because her daughter had Down syndrome. They [the family] taught me that expectations make a difference. They look at all the positive gains their daughter has made. Their attitude has made a difference in their daughter's progress.

The way a student presents his or her family's "message" is often a telling sign of how powerful the home visit can be.

An experience with a family whose child was born prematurely gave one of the medical students a chance to speculate on a similar outcome for other children.

I visited a family whose child was born at twenty-three weeks. Some of these kids are born so premature you begin to wonder, Are we doing anyone any good by keeping these twenty-three-, twenty-four-, twenty-five-week-old kids alive? And I was under the assumption that these kids would never have any quality of life. . . . It [the home visit] was amazing. It made me feel a lot better about the neonatal intensive care nursery and some of these premature kids, to see this kid five years down the road. I'm assuming others will do as well!

The opportunity to reflect on the home visits is critical to the Medical Education Project learning experience. And the physicians associated with Parent to Parent have been facilitating these discussions since the project began. Each exchange is yet another occasion to reinforce the family perspective. For example, a student made this remark when talking about the home visit:

What struck me the most was that it's not the big things but the little things that are taken away from the parents, freedom-wise. I didn't know how much was at stake: the loss of personal freedoms.

This lesson, powerful in itself, is confirmed by Dr. Swartz:

We narrow the problem to something we can work with. We look at one piece of the fabric, not the whole fabric. Our system of handling these problems and the family's way of dealing with problems are quite different, and we need to be constantly reminded.

CONCLUSION

Families and physicians working together inspired the creation and influenced the success of the Medical Education Project. As explained by three social analysts at the University of Vermont,

Families and professionals bring essential knowledge, skills, and experience to a collaborative relationship. In the past, families were often considered the receivers of professional expertise, without acknowledgement of the unique and valuable contribution they make. The collaborative model recognized the expertise of all the people involved in caring for a child with special [health] needs. (Bishop, Wall & Arango, 1993, p. 20)

This is truly a collaborative model—an example of how the collective wisdom and experience of families and physicians can expand and intensify the education of medical students. According to a recent article in the *Journal of Pediatrics*,

> More needs to be learned about the value system of physicians and how they develop caring attitudes about parental needs. Medical education is generally oriented toward teaching factual and objective material, with less emphasis on emotional and sociocultural content. What factors influence medical students' and residents' abilities to communicate in a caring manner? Are physicians convinced by their training that parental perspectives have importance and can help educate clinicians? (Sharp, Strauss & Lorch, 1992)

The Medical Education Project was designed with these questions in mind. We are confident that this model of medical education will continue to generate caring, compassionate physicians and will advance the "art" of practicing medicine.

Plans are presently under way to offer pediatric residents at the University of Vermont College of Medicine an opportunity to have an extended, one-to-three-year relationship with a family. Most recently, the University of Vermont School of Nursing has requested that a home visit experience be required of each undergraduate in the nursing program. This expansion of the Medical Education Project will extend its impact by producing even more medical professionals with a better understanding of the families they serve.

NOTE

1. Special thanks to each of the forty-two families who have opened their homes and hearts to more than 493 medical students since the beginning of the Medical Education Project.

REFERENCES

Bishop, K. K., Wall, J., & Arango, P. (1993). *Family/professional collaboration for children with special health needs and their families*. Burlington: Department of Social Work, University of Vermont.

Sharp, M. C., Strauss, R. P., & Lorch, S. C. (1992). Communicating medical bad news: Parents' experiences and preferences. *Journal of Pediatrics* 121:539–546.

7

Graduate Medical Education in Pediatrics: Preparing Reliable Allies for Parents of Children with Special Health Care Needs

W. Carl Cooley

In 1978, the *Future of Pediatric Education* was published as a Task Force Report of the American Academy of Pediatrics (Task Force on Pediatric Education, 1978). A sample of seven thousand pediatricians was surveyed regarding their thoughts about the adequacy of their pediatric training as preparation for the realities of pediatric practice. Among the most notable areas of underemphasis in training identified in this survey were the biosocial and developmental aspects of pediatrics. The pediatricians also felt ill-prepared in the areas of community pediatrics, handicapping conditions and chronic illness, and medical ethics. The report recommended that training programs greatly expand their emphasis on the biosocial aspects of pediatric care.

Fifteen years have passed since the publication of the *Future of Pediatric Education.* The future is now! This chapter reviews broadly and with specific examples how contemporary pediatric training programs are correcting the deficiencies identified in the 1978 report and how well these training programs are meeting the newer challenges of the 1980s and 1990s. The structure of a typical pediatric residency curriculum is discussed in light of some of the forces that shape areas of emphasis and omission. Portions of the research literature about pediatric training since the 1978 Task Force Report are reviewed. Finally, a number of examples describe how values such as family-centered care, parent–professional partnerships, and cross-disciplinary collaboration are being incorporated into training. The hope is to familiarize the nonmedical reader with the nature of pediatric postgraduate education, while providing all readers with insights about current trends and future directions for pediatric training.

PEDIATRICIANS AS RELIABLE ALLIES

Families of children with special health care needs provide the very greatest portion of their children's direct care and must become skillful advocates and service coordinators. Even with the help of the most accessible and well-organized systems of formal support, successful families also identify and utilize their own informal support systems. For many families, these informal support systems may be characterized as a network of reliable alliances. Spouses and other family members are natural reliable allies, but others may include friends, neighbors, pastoral counselors, school bus drivers, librarians, and many others. Among the formal or professional sources of support, skillful families quickly learn to distinguish the reliable allies from the less dependable or helpful resources among teachers, doctors, family support providers, case managers, and early intervention providers.

Families find that reliable allies are

- *experienced*—They have knowledge or expertise that is needed; have been through similar experiences and are familiar with similar issues.
- *dependable*—They are accessible; return phone calls; are there when needed.
- *unconditionally supportive*—They are on the family's side; are not judgmental; trust and believe parents; tolerate disagreement.
- *comfortable with feelings*—They validate family members' feelings and do not minimize them; are not patronizing; are open to full range of feelings.
- *reciprocating*—They share values; use and share personal experiences; make the family feel less alone.

In order to train future pediatricians to be more reliable as allies in working with families, methods are needed that address the requirements of a reliable alliance. These requirements, then, are mutual respect, mutual trust, common goals and visions, a sharing of information, and a shared stake in the outcomes whether good or bad. Pediatricians who are unable to infuse the parent–professional relationship with these elements are not likely to be regarded as reliable allies by parents dealing with complex and demanding issues in their children. Such a pediatrician may still be regarded as knowledgeable or capable in the technical aspects of care, but families will look elsewhere for sources of reliable support. As we examine ideas and models for increasing the family- and community-centeredness of pediatric training, we should consider how well each model encourages the development of the characteristics described above.

PEDIATRIC RESIDENCY TRAINING

Medical students who express an interest in pediatrics may have elective opportunities for pediatric experiences prior to graduation, beyond the basic courses taken by all students. Unfortunately, during the 1980s a steady decline in interest in pediatric or other primary health care careers was evident among medical students (Council on Graduate Medical Education, 1990). A variety of pressures—not the least of which, financial—seemed to be motivating students toward specialized, often technical, and usually more highly paid fields of medicine. The accumulation of large student-loan debts contributed to the perception that one's career should enable one to repay these loans quickly. Another prominent concern voiced by students was job satisfaction: Would pediatric practice be sufficiently challenging, interesting, and varied to provide an ongoing source of personal gratification and intellectual stimulation throughout a career? Many hospital-based training programs located largely in tertiary medical centers did little to provide a role model of the best practices in primary care and tended to convey the impression that specialization was the path to excellence. The issue of student loans cannot be resolved here, but hopefully changes in the organization of our health care system will address training to the extent that students are no longer selecting careers based on income potential. However, job interest and satisfaction could be enhanced considerably if pediatricians-in-training were provided the skills needed to make a community-based primary care practice a lively home for medical, information, and coordination services for all the children and families in the community (Sia, 1992).

Pediatric residency is typically a three-year experiential training process that follows directly upon the four years of medical school training. Completion of an approved pediatric residency followed by a pediatric specialty board examination is required for a physician to become "board certified" in pediatrics. The bylaws of most hospitals require this board certification for a pediatric physician to become a member of the hospital's staff. If a pediatrician desires further training in a pediatric subspecialty such as cardiology, neonatology, or endocrinology, additional years beyond the pediatric residency are required.

In many teaching centers, pediatric residents are employed by the hospital to provide much of the direct care in the hospital's inpatient and outpatient settings under the supervision of fully trained and experienced "staff" or "attending" pediatricians. Pediatric residents are "real doctors" in that they have completed their M.D. degree and are licensed to practice at least within the confines of their training program. The teaching hospitals in which they work depend on them as a relatively inexpensive source of labor to deliver many of the hospitals' direct care services. The consequence of this working relationship with the hospital is pressure on the residency programs to "cover" or staff the pediatrics ward, the newborn intensive care unit, the pediatric intensive care unit, the emergency room, and the various outpatient clinics. This coverage requirement in many settings takes priority over activities away from the hospital, out in the community with families or community-based professionals.

Residency programs are also subject to the credentialing requirements of their national accreditation boards, which set the standards for pediatric residency curricula and then review the adherence of each program to those standards. While standards in the past allowed considerable elective opportunity and emphasized residents' participation in outreach programs and other community-based activities, there has recently been more emphasis on in-hospital, direct care–based experiences in the intensive care units, the emergency room, and the clinics of subspecialties such as cardiology and hematology/oncology. Accreditation is a force that can make more difficult any curricular revision in the direction of family-oriented care. On the other hand, it is a potential arena in which to focus pressure for change so that the notions of partnerships in care, service coordination, family support and empowerment, and community-based care are regarded as curriculum elements of equal importance to the more traditional and technical aspects of care.

RESIDENCY TRAINING SINCE THE TASK FORCE REPORT

By 1984, one survey reported that 49 percent of residency programs had incorporated formal behavioral pediatrics training into their pediatric residencies, with an additional 38 percent of programs offering some behavioral training. Thirteen percent of programs offered no exposure to behavioral pediatrics (Zebal & Friedman, 1984). Another survey in the same year found few major changes since the 1978 Task Force Report except for increased continuity experience and more mandatory experience in child psychiatry and behavioral pediatrics (Weinberger & Oski, 1984). More recently, Wender, Bijur, and Boyce (1992) surveyed a sample of three thousand pediatricians who completed their residency training after 1978, using an almost identical survey instrument as that used in the 1978 Task Force Report. This study showed relatively little change in the high numbers of pediatricians who perceived that they had received insufficient training in similar areas as in the 1978 report. More than 50 percent of those surveyed considered their training inadequate in such areas as psychosocial and behavior problems, mental retardation, and learning disabilities. On the other hand, pediatricians who had trained in the second half of the first ten-year period after the 1978 Task Force Report noted improvements in exposure to developmental and behavioral pediatrics. Two-thirds of the group that had trained after 1984 also noted that their training was sufficient in the areas of interviewing and counseling.

Absent from these surveys is any information about training exposure to the issues of families. Such exposure ideally would include both the academic study of research about family systems, family stress and support, and families' adaptations to having a child with special needs, as well as the utilization of families and other consumers as teachers regarding their experiences, their knowledge about their children, and their expectations of health care providers.

Between 10 percent and 20 percent of children are affected by chronic conditions associated either with illness or with disability (Gortmaker & Sappenfield, 1984). When that fact is combined with the results of the surveys described above in which pediatricians-in-practice perceive that their training has not adequately prepared them for dealing with the biosocial, developmental, and behavioral aspects of care, it is surprising to find that published guidelines for training still do not promote correcting the deficiencies. The Ambulatory Pediatric Association, for example, has published *Educational Guidelines for Training in General/Ambulatory Pediatrics* (Education Committee of the Ambulatory Pediatric Association, 1984). This document is an extensive, itemized review of all that should be included in the training of both medical students and pediatric residents in ambulatory pediatrics. Though it speaks of the need to develop "good communication skills," there is no mention of parent–professional partnership, mutual respect, knowledge about family dynamics, promoting self-care skills in children with chronic illness, or collaborating with other community professionals. There is no mention of knowledge about early intervention services, family support systems, or case management. The need for pediatricians to prepare for a leadership role in the organization of services at the community level is not addressed. The learning methods described in this document are limited to didactic sessions (conferences, lectures, and seminars), texts (books and journals), audiovisual materials, and patients (practical experiences in the clinic and hospital or role-playing situations). Specific references to children and families as teachers—or other than in their role as patients—are not to be found.

In the late 1980s, with a grant from the U.S. Department of Education, a national task force of developmental and behavioral pediatricians and other experts was assembled with the goal of ensuring "that pediatric residents in all accredited programs . . . receive effective and comprehensive training in developmental pediatrics" (Guralnick et al., 1987, p. 3). Among other things, this task force developed for residents a comprehensive curriculum in developmental pediatrics. This curriculum covered ten broad noncategorical units of study ranging from knowledge of handicapping conditions to interdisciplinary process and team functioning, attitudes toward handicapping conditions, and community service systems. It included extensive reading materials and suggestions about teaching methods. In addition, the overall project offered training in the use of the curriculum and undertook an evaluation by surveying a total of 160 residents at fifteen different training sites. The evaluation involved a comparison of residents who had been exposed to the curriculum with others who had not. On both subjective and objective measures, the curriculum was found to be highly effective in preparing residents to address the needs of children with developmental disabilities and their families.

INNOVATIONS IN PEDIATRIC RESIDENCY TRAINING—MODEL EXAMPLES

Redefinition of the role of the primary care physician in the care of children with disabilities and with complex health care needs continues to evolve. Descriptions during the past decade have identified a number of newly recognized responsibilities: screening and identification of developmental differences; appropriate referrals to medical and nonmedical resources; regular, accessible communication with families; connecting families with needed community resources; and providing a service coordination role for health care services (Martin, 1985). Added to this list might be such concerns as the enhancement of self-care skills among older children with chronic health care concerns, the participation of families as partners not only in the individual office encounter but in an advisory capacity to the pediatric office as a whole, and the pediatrician's leadership role in the community as one of the important resources for children and families (Cooley, in press).

Pediatric residents receive ample exposure to hospitalized children with disabilities and special health care needs. In fact, residents' experiences in this regard may color their views of such children and their families. There may be a tendency to view life for such children as an endless sequence of hospitalizations, and their families as living under a steady state of stress and demoralization. Residents may not experience that families do return to a day-to-day mode of functioning, nor are they likely to see other children and families for whom hospitalizations are rarely if ever necessary. Residents should either venture into the communities where children and families live, or else the families and other members of those communities (teachers, primary physicians, child care providers) must be invited to the medical center as valued teachers for the residents about the "rest of the story" for children with special health care needs.

Dartmouth–Hitchcock Medical Center

The Dartmouth–Hitchcock Medical Center in Lebanon, New Hampshire, provides an example of a program offering residents and medical students insights into the challenges and accomplishments of families of children with special health care needs. Each pediatric resident and each medical student during his or her third-year pediatric rotation is required to provide respite care on at least one occasion for a family with a child who has a disability or a chronic illness. These encounters are organized through a local parent-directed family support organization, which maintains a roster of families interested in participating in the project. The respite care experience is preceded by a get-acquainted visit between the pediatric resident or medical student and the family during which the respite care is planned. The student or resident is expected to provide at least six hours of respite care, following which a second interview with the family takes place. Soon after the respite care experience, a debriefing session is held with a pediatric staff member.

Most residents and students find this program to be a valuable and enlightening experience in spite of the need to give up an evening or weekend day. In many cases, an ongoing relationship has evolved in which additional respite care or other meetings with the families take place. Currently, plans are in progress for the respite care relationship to evolve into a service coordination and family support role on a longitudinal basis during the residents' entire three-year training program.

Residents are also provided a series of exposures to community-based services in early intervention, preschool special education in natural environments, childcare programs, and family support organizations. The residents are expected to serve as nonvoting ex-officio board members of community-based nonprofit organizations that serve families or provide community-based services.

A number of other medical centers have developed similar programs for medical students and/or pediatric residents in order to enhance their understanding and application of the principles of family-centered care (DiVenere, Frankowski & Stifler, 1991).

University of Maryland

At the University of Maryland, the Division of Behavioral and Developmental Pediatrics has developed a comprehensive training program for pediatric residents to provide experiences in the care of children with disabilities and other special health care needs. The goals of this program are as follows: (1) to develop a comprehensive knowledge base regarding the medical and developmental issues of children with chronic disabilities and their treatment; (2) to understand the principles of family-centered care; (3) to be knowledgeable about community resources available to children with disabilities and their families; (4) to develop comfort and expertise in interdisciplinary settings; and (5) to understand the team process. These goals are met through integrated teaching strategies in two mandatory rotations as well as ongoing exposure to "developmental rounds" in the newborn intensive care unit and the regular pediatric inpatient unit. Off-site or outreach experiences are provided through structured observations in childcare settings, with home visits by a community health nurse, at developmental medicine consultations in a school setting, and through a visit to a specialized school setting for children experiencing blindness. In addition, role-play and videotaping techniques are used to focus on the development of interviewing skills and sensitive approaches to "breaking diagnostic news" to parents and families (Wachtel et al., 1992).

St. Christopher's Children's Hospital

At St. Christopher's Children's Hospital in Philadelphia, a similar program is aimed at helping pediatric residents to acquire the skills necessary to join parents in their effort to meet the comprehensive care requirements of their children experiencing special health care needs. The project has included the development of a computerized resource directory providing pediatric residents with direct access to community-based resources and referral options for children and families. A second element of this project involves a structured exposure to several exemplary early intervention programs in their community settings (Fee, 1992).

University of North Carolina

The Community Outreach Training Program at the University of North Carolina School of Medicine was instituted in the early 1980s, partially in response to the findings of the 1978 Task Force Report (Sharp & Lorch, 1988). The objectives of this program were to increase student and resident skills in these areas: (1) knowledge of various domains of development; (2) understanding of the complex influences of environment on growth and development; (3) evaluating and managing behavioral and developmental problems; (4) awareness of nonmedical resources for children and families; (5) ability to communicate with professionals in nonmedical disciplines, and with parents, to promote better service coordination; (6) awareness of the ethical issues associated with health care delivery; and (7) self-awareness of their own attitudes and emotional reactions to clinical and educational experiences. The program does not strive to "take pediatric expertise out to the community; rather it reaches out for the community's help in teaching trainees" (Sharp & Lorch, 1988, p. 317).

The UNC program is built around four one-month modules: normal early-childhood development; disorders of development in early childhood; normal school-age and adolescent development; and disorders in development in the older child and adolescent. Each module combines knowledge-base and skills development with exposure to relevant community-based agencies and services. A total of twenty-five community agencies were utilized to provide settings for the outreach curriculum. Though this program was developed under a grant from the National Fund for Medical Education, evaluations of its effectiveness—and its popularity with residents and students—have led to ongoing departmental funding for a program coordinator, and to the permanent inclusion of the Community Outreach Training Program into the residency training curriculum.

Michigan State University

The Chronic Illness Teaching Program was established in 1984 by the Department of Pediatrics and Human Development in the College of Human Medicine at Michigan State University (Desguin, 1988). The aims of this program are to prepare the resident to be a provider of continuity of care, a coordinator of care, an educator, an advocate, and a counselor. The program spans all three years of pediatric residency training and has four major components: (1) family studies; (2) services for children with special health care needs; (3) knowledge and skills; and (4) issues of chronic illness. All four components are incorporated into a month-long rotation in each of the three years of training.

Family studies is considered the key area of focus for the program. In this component, every one of the residents must undertake a longitudinal family study each year, based on at least one extended home interview with the family of a child with special health care needs. The resident also accompanies the family to a variety of visits to health or social service agencies, observes the child at school, and interviews other professionals involved in providing services to the family. A literature review of research about families is conducted, focusing on areas prompted by the resident's experience with the family. In the third year, each resident makes a final presentation of what has been learned through this longitudinal, qualitative study. The other three components of the program's curriculum are addressed with similar combinations of outreach experiences and readings supervised by the mentoring of faculty members.

In evaluations of this project, its organizers asked the first thirteen participants how likely it was they would be caring for children with complex health care needs as practicing pediatricians. Eight of the eleven respondents indicated that the teaching program had made them more likely to assume a larger role in the care of such children. The organizers found three factors, in particular, that were important to the program's success: first, the creation of "protected time" for residents during their chronic-illness rotation, to avoid competing with the demands of other rotations and of the "night-call schedule"; second, enough flexibility to allow each resident to study an area of chronic illness or disability of particular interest to him or her; and third, a requirement for long-term contact on the family's own turf, away from the medical setting.

SUMMARY

In 1988, a survey was conducted of all U.S. pediatric residency training programs, inquiring about the utilization of community-based sites for resident education (Alpert et al., 1991). The survey listed twenty-one generic community sites ranging from private pediatric-practice offices to schools, early intervention programs, courts, and childcare centers. Responses were received from 200 out of the 237 programs surveyed. Among the most frequently used sites were private physicians' offices (81.5% of the programs having indicated use), "crippled children's services" (56%), neighborhood health centers (65%), rehabilitation centers (52%), and child protection agencies (52%). In general, the study showed extensive use of a wide range of community-based sites. The survey failed to inquire about contact with families, about home visits, or about the nature of the exposure to community sites. However, this survey—along with the selection of examples described in this chapter—provides some indication that a more widespread movement is occurring in pediatric residency training to address some of the deficiencies identified in the 1978 Task Force Report and, more importantly, to prepare pediatricians for roles as reliable allies to families of children with special health care needs as they face the challenges of the 1990s and beyond.

REFERENCES

Alpert, J. J., Blodgett, F. M., Gargas, D. C., Jenkins, R., Kaplan, D. W., Kohrt, A., Levine, G., & O'Hare, D. (1991). A survey of community (out-of-hospital) sites used in pediatric training. *Pediatrics* 87:719–721.

Cooley, W. C. (in press). Community outreach—extending and enhancing care where families live. In S. L. Hostler, ed., *Family-centered care: An approach to implementation.* Washington, DC: U.S. Department of Health and Human Services.

Council on Graduate Medical Education. (1990). *Reform in medical education and medical education in the ambulatory setting.* Publication No. HRSA-P-DM-91-4. Washington, DC: U.S. Department of Health and Human Services.

Desguin, B. W. (1988, February). Preparing pediatric residents for the primary care of children with chronic illness and their families: The chronic illness teaching program. *Zero to Three*, pp. 7–10.

DiVenere, N., Frankowski, B., & Stifler, D. (1991). The Medical Education Project: A shared learning experience incorporating the principles of family-centered care in physician education. *Medical Home Newsletter* 4:2–7.

Education Committee of the Ambulatory Pediatric Association. (1984). *Educational guidelines for training in general/ambulatory pediatrics.* McLean, VA: Ambulatory Pediatrics Association.

Fee, M. (1992). Parent–physician partnership: A tripartite approach to resident education. In R. B. Darling & M. I. Peter, eds., *Creating family–professional partnerships: Educating physicians and other health professionals to care for children with chronic and disabling conditions.* Conference proceedings. Honolulu: Hawaii Medical Association.

Gortmaker, S., & Sappenfield, W. (1984). Chronic childhood disorders: Prevalence and impact. *Pediatric Clinics of North America* 31:3–18.

Guralnick, M. J., Bennett, F. C., Heiser, K. E., & Richardson, H. B. (1987). Training future primary care pediatricians to serve handicapped children and their families. *Topics in Early Childhood Special Education* 6:1–11.

Martin, E. W. (1985). Pediatrician's role in the care of disabled children. *Pediatrics in Review* 6:275–281.

Sharp, M. C., & Lorch, S. C. (1988). A community outreach training program for pediatric residents and medical students. *Journal of Medical Education* 63:316–322.

Sia, C. C. J. (1992). Medical home and child advocacy in the 1990's. *Pediatrics* 90:419–423.

Task Force on Pediatric Education. (1978). *The future of pediatric education.* Washington, DC: American Academy of Pediatrics.

Wachtel, R. C., Grossman, L., Hyman, S. L., & Kappelman, M. (1992). Helping future pediatricians to know and understand: Preservice education for professionals who care for children with chronic and disabling conditions. In R. B. Darling & M. I. Peter, eds., *Creating family–professional partnerships: Educating physicians and other health professionals to care for children with chronic and disabling conditions.* Conference proceedings. Honolulu: Hawaii Medical Association.

Weinberger, H. L., & Oski, F. A. (1984). A survey of pediatric resident training programs 5 years after the Task Force Report. *Pediatrics* 74:523–526.

Wender, E. H., Bijur, P. E., & Boyce, W. T. (1992). Pediatric residency training: Ten years after the Task Force Report. *Pediatrics* 90:876–880.

Zebal, B. H., & Friedman, S. B. (1984). A nationwide survey of behavioral pediatric residency training. *Journal of Developmental and Behavioral Pediatrics* 5:331–335.

CONTINUING EDUCATION MODELS

8

Preparing Physicians through Continuing Medical Education

Margo I. Peter
and
Calvin C. J. Sia

The morbidity of children has changed and the problems threatening children today include a host of developmental and behavioral problems in addition to the "old" morbidities of illness and disease. This changing morbidity compels a corresponding change in the way primary care physicians are trained to treat children.

Green and Haggerty (1990) chose adaptation as the unifying theme for their recent text on ambulatory pediatrics. In it, they promote the idea that helping children and parents adapt and cope is a vital and necessary part of the continuum of pediatric care. Furthermore, they encourage primary care physicians to establish bridges between the biologic, psychological, developmental, and sociocultural aspects of child health and to incorporate this into their traditional roles of prevention, health promotion, treatment, and rehabilitation. Thus, helping families adapt to changes requires that physicians themselves adapt to a more comprehensive way of thinking about their role as caregivers.

In order to be responsive to the changing needs of families, we must first remember that families are the ultimate consumers of health care. Therefore, families should be at the center of the service delivery systems designed to serve them, and family-centered care must be the driving philosophy of our developing systems. We must further recognize that the multiple and pervasive nature of the risk factors challenging children today require collaborative relationships among the providers of health, education, and human services. Thus we must become active advocates for a well-integrated network of services addressing the total needs of the child and family. Incorporating the "medical home" into these integrated service delivery systems is critical to assuring comprehensive services.

According to the American Academy of Pediatrics (1992), a medical home should encompass the following services:

1. Provision of preventive care including—but not restricted to—immunizations, growth and development assessments, appropriate screening, health care supervision, and patient and parental counseling about health and psycho-social issues.
2. Assurance of ambulatory and inpatient care for acute illnesses, twenty-four hours a day, seven days a week—during the working day, after hours, on weekends, fifty-two weeks a year.
3. Provision of care over an extended period of time to enhance continuity.
4. Identification of the need for subspecialty consultation and referrals—and knowing from whom and where these can be obtained. Provision of medical information about the patient to the consultant. Evaluation of the consultant's recommendations, implementation of recommendations that are indicated and appropriate, and interpretation of these to the family.
5. Interaction with school and community agencies to be certain that special health needs of the individual child are addressed.
6. Maintenance of central record and data base containing all pertinent medical information about the child, including information about hospitalizations. This record should be accessible, but confidentiality must be assured.

The challenge for physicians is to provide a true medical home for all children in their communities, in order to supply an ongoing source for continuous, comprehensive, coordinated health care (Brewer et al., 1989, p. 1058). This is a tall order and a considerable task.

Making the medical home a reality for all children requires, first, legislative policy to assure funding for and access to services; second, public–private coordination to assure availability of services; and third, physician education and training to enhance skills and awareness. Primary care physicians interested in providing optimal care to children with special needs should equip themselves with the knowledge, skills, and resources necessary to do so.

Where should this training begin? Ideally, such training should be integrated into all levels of training including medical school, residency training, and continuing medical education (CME). Today there are many innovative programs, such as those outlined in previous chapters. Unfortunately, these are the exception rather than the rule, though, and most are recent additions to traditional training curriculums. Many mature clinicians received little or no such training in the new morbidity. That it is a felt need among practicing physicians is clearly illustrated in Chapter 10 of this volume. In meeting this need, CME training is the best—and perhaps only—way to reach the large number of physicians already in practice.

Hawaii has been at the forefront of efforts to promote CME training in the care of children with special needs. Six years ago, with the support of the Office of Maternal and Child Health, we piloted a series of CME trainings in an effort to promote physician involvement with these children. A year later we formalized the training into a CME curriculum for the practicing physician: "The Pediatrician and the New Morbidity." This chapter will review that curriculum, as well as provide a summary of several other innovative CME programs.

THE PEDIATRICIAN AND THE NEW MORBIDITY

The Hawaiian CME program is designed to assist primary care physicians in developing an awareness of the importance of medical homes for children with special needs, as well as to provide the insight, awareness, and skills for providing such care. The CME program is presented as a series of three small group meetings ("modules"). Each session is approximately two hours long, and active participation is encouraged. Training is accomplished with a team of trainers that includes physicians, parents, and a facilitator. A brief mention of what the training is *not* is perhaps in order before we discuss the specifics of what it is.

It is not just for pediatricians. Granted, the title suggests that the materials are applicable only to pediatricians. This is unfortunate and inaccurate. Most children in Hawaii have pediatricians as their primary care physicians (PMDs); hence our emphasis on that group. However, many children elsewhere receive primary care from family practitioners, and the material is equally relevant for those physicians. We strongly promote the involvement of family practitioners in such training and encourage those interested in implementing CME training to collaborate with their local chapters of the American Academy of Pediatrics (AAP) and American Academy of Family Practice (AAFP).

The material in "The Pediatrician and the New Morbidity" was not designed to transform primary care physicians into disability specialists. It was designed to provide broad constructs, which can be applied to improve care for the gamut of children with special needs. The goal was to challenge old beliefs about children with special needs and to begin a dialogue among physicians, community providers, and families about what defines optimal care for these children.

At the heart of the training is former Surgeon General Dr. C. Everett Koop's call for community-based, coordinated, family-centered care. Accordingly, the training is comprised of three modules: Module I, The PMD and Community-based Care; Module II, The PMD and Coordinated Care; and Module III, the PMD and Family-centered Care.

Module I: The PMD and Community-based Care

The first session focuses on the role of the PMD in providing a medical home for children. A practicing physician functions as the trainer, accompanied by an early intervention service provider. The concepts of the medical home and the new morbidity are defined and discussed. In addition to these concepts, the three elements of family-centered, community-based, and coordinated care are introduced and related to the medical home.

Emphasis is on the critical role of the PMD in early detection of developmental problems, and PMDs are encouraged to integrate a developmental focus into their regular well-child care. Several screening tools are examined and demonstrated. Four key elements of effective screening are discussed: (1) awareness of the child and family's medical history; (2) physical examination; (3) parental observations and concerns; and (4) use of formal screening tools. It is stressed that elimination or inappropriate application of any of these components will negatively impact the effectiveness of the screening process. The importance of early intervention is outlined, as well as the valuable role of the PMD as an access point for early intervention services.

Module II: The PMD and Coordinated Care

The second session emphasizes the need for collaboration between medical homes and other community service providers. The training team includes a group facilitator and practicing physician. Participants in this session include physicians from the target community as well as representatives from community agencies serving children with special needs. The session begins with an outline of the benefits of and barriers to coordination among the myriad of providers in any given community. Medical case management is differentiated from overall case management (care coordination), and the role of the physician in care coordination is discussed. Emphasis is placed on choosing the appropriate care coordinator based on a child's unique needs and family preference.

Networking is the primary function of this meeting, and participants spend the bulk of their time familiarizing themselves with each other and the services each has to offer. The focus on networking evolved as we realized that a first critical step in developing collaborative relationships between PMDs and community agencies was getting acquainted. We found that few of our participants had enjoyed the opportunity to do this previously. Anecdotal evidence suggested that this simple strategy has led to more and varied referrals by physicians to community agencies.

Module III: The PMD and Family-centered Care

We consider the third session to be the heart and soul of the CME modules, and it is often the most well-received. The overarching theme is parent–professional partnership, and the training team is comprised of a parent and a physician. The idea of family-centered care is presented as a growing philosophy of health care, heralding a system of service delivery that will be more flexible, accessible, and responsive to families. The point is made that clinical success turns on how well we clinicians incorporate the family into our system of care. Physicians are encouraged to adopt a family-centered style, which may require a new way of doing things and a willingness to listen, support, and respond to families. Emphasis is placed on the fact that the goal has changed from solving families' problems *for* them to helping *them* deal more effectively with those problems.

Two topics are discussed in depth. The first is the issue of sharing diagnostic news; and the second is the formation of lasting partnerships with parents in order to enhance the care provided and improve the outcomes for their children. As to the first topic, sharing diagnostic news with families puts a unique stress on the relationship between PMD and patient. Unfortunately, little or no formal training in accomplishing this difficult task is provided by a traditional medical education. For this reason, concrete suggestions about the dos-and-don'ts of sharing diagnostic news are given during the session. Emphasis is placed on sharing complete information, the demystification of medical jargon, and parental empowerment in decision making. Issues in sharing diagnostic news are also discussed in Chapters 4 and 9. As to the second topic, the parent–professional partnership is stressed in this module, and four key elements of such a partnership are identified: information; support; access to services; and respect. Physicians are encouraged to form alliances with parents in order to maximize their effectiveness.

The real value of this session lies in the training team. The physician and the parent each model their message as they take turns sharing information with the participants. The physician trainer provides clinically specific examples and is able to relate frustrations and difficulties unique to her role as a physician. The parent trainer serves as a window into the experience of parents during the diagnostic process. This provides a rare opportunity for physicians to see things from the consumer's side and to ask sensitive questions without the risk of hurting a patient's feelings.

ADDITIONAL STRATEGIES

Just as treatment strategies for children and families must be developed based on individual needs, so too the strategies used to implement CME training must be tailored to fit the unique situation of each individual community of physicians. Several variations in methodology have been tried with success, and they are outlined briefly below.

Train-the-Trainers Model

A train-the-trainers model can maximize funding dollars while minimizing problems related to geographical expanse. Florida's Institute for Child Health Policy, in collaboration with the University of Miami's Mailman Center for Child Development, received funding from the Florida Department of Education to implement a CME training program that would foster family-centered care for children eligible for services under Part H of Public Law (P.L.) 99-457. From the outset, key players were invited to collaborate on planning and implementation—including physicians, parents, and public health program administrators. A parent was chosen to serve as overall coordinator for the project.

Parent and physician trainers were chosen from nineteen identified districts of the state. A total of seventeen physician–parent teams participated in a weekend train-the-trainer workshop. During these sessions, the teams received training about family-centered care, developmental screening, and early intervention policy and services. In addition, they were presented with information regarding adult learning and suggested strategies for conducting local training sessions for parents, physicians, and early intervention professionals. Objectives for the weekend sessions were as follows: (1) to provide physicians and parents with an overview of early intervention initiatives; (2) to recommend and demonstrate developmentally appropriate tools for screening and identifying children with special needs; (3) to prepare physicians and parents to act as agents of change in the local community; (4) to prepare physicians and parents to form partnerships in the practice of family-centered care; and (5) to provide content for training modules as well as strategies for implementing training sessions. Training teams were asked to conduct at least one session in their home community and were provided a stipend for doing so. Out of a possible nineteen teams, twelve completed their mission, and a total of 123 physicians, 86 parents, and 95 other professionals attended training in their home communities.

Several advantages and disadvantages to the train-the-trainer approach were noted by project organizers (Siderits et al., 1992). There was significant variability in the number of participants per session. Sessions conducted in large medical centers where physicians attended routine CME programs, and those whose trainers invested time and energy to personally recruit prospective participants, had the largest audiences. There was also variability in the degree of "teamwork" reflected by the training teams. A few teams were dominated by physicians; and the planners felt that more emphasis needed to be placed on parents' expertise as trainers, and more time allotted for training teams to establish rapport. The organizers reported these additional lessons as well: (1) The health care providers needed additional time and practice using developmental screening techniques; (2) CME credits proved to be strong enticements for physician attendance; (3) verbal or telephone follow-up and recruitment are necessary to assure participation; (4) a meticulous and motivated project coordinator is a necessity; and (5) pre-workshop sessions with physician trainers should be conducted to reduce anxiety and increase the likelihood of collaboration between parents and physicians.

The project successfully trained more than three hundred physicians, parents, and other professionals and is planning to follow up with written self-study materials and additional sessions for allied health care providers.

Large Group/Grand Rounds Format

Another effective strategy for CME training involves using existing formats to disseminate important information. Two notable examples of this are efforts initiated by the Arizona Chapter of the American Academy of Pediatrics and the Medical College of Ohio.

In Arizona, a unique partnership was formed between the state's Interagency Coordinating Council (ICC) and the AAP chapter to accomplish training aimed at ensuring that every child who has, or is at risk of having, a disability be identified and treated appropriately (Melmed, 1991).

Collaboration was identified as essential for all levels of planning and implementation. Representatives from the Arizona Chapter of the AAP and the Office of Maternal and Child Health invited experts from pediatrics, speech and language pathology, audiology, occupational therapy, the Division of Developmental Disabilities (DDD), and parents to review and refine training materials.

The training team was comprised of a pediatrician and representatives from Pilot Parent Partnerships and the DDD. Thus, the team itself served as a collaborative model. Training sessions were one and a half hours in length and were conducted initially in small groups. As a result of the positive response, the training team then decided to expand its network.

In a statewide survey, twenty pediatricians indicated a willingness to serve as trainers. A two-day seminar was conducted for potential trainers. Content included an overview of P.L. 99-457 and the physician's role, a discussion of issues related to early identification, parents' perspectives regarding the importance of the physician to the family, the need for sensitivity when sharing a diagnosis, and an overview of local resources available to physicians.

The training teams made presentations to groups of pediatricians, osteopaths, and family practitioners at dinner meetings, grand rounds, hospital meetings, and conferences. In all, more than 650 health care professionals attended trainings in twenty sites throughout the state. Training organizers followed up with two newsletters containing related information. The success of the effort was considered largely to be the result of the collaborative nature of the effort as well as the manner of presentation. Organizers recommend that material be presented in an authoritative manner, be exciting, and presented in such a way as to be perceived by listeners as useful to them in the future. Brevity and variety were also considered important for sustained attention!

In Ohio in 1990, the Department of Pediatrics of the Medical College of Ohio initiated a CME program funded by the Early Intervention Unit of the Ohio Department of Health (Rupert, 1991). The goal: to familiarize pediatricians, family physicians, and their office nursing staff with P.L. 99-457 and Ohio's plan for implementing it. Curricular objectives were to positively affect the attitudes and knowledge of these professionals, their role in identifying and caring for children with special health needs, and the roles of agencies and groups in serving these children and families.

Co-sponsorship was arranged with the Ohio chapters of the AAP and AAFP. Meetings were convened at a local hospital and scheduled in place of regularly held hospital-based CME programs or in conjunction with a regional pediatric society meeting. Program announcements and articles were published in the quarterly newsletters for the local AAP and AAFP. All programs were free of charge and were approved for continuing medical and nursing education accreditation. Program attendees were encouraged to preregister, and self-study packets were mailed to each registrant prior to the meetings.

A three-hour training program was implemented in seven different cities by a training team that included a pediatrician, an early intervention specialist, and a parent. A practicing pediatrician in the targeted community was invited to serve as a local coordinator and decided the best date, time, and location. Two members of the training team were specific to each community. A parent and an early intervention specialist were recruited from the target community, and this helped assure relevance and immediacy. More than two hundred people attended the training conferences, two-thirds of whom were physicians. The partnership developed at that time between the Ohio Department of Health and the Ohio chapters of the AAP and AAFP continues, and additional training activities are planned.

Direct Mail

A direct mail campaign has the advantage of reaching those physicians who can't be enticed to leave their office for a formal CME session. The Minnesota chapters of the AAP and AAFP's newsletter, entitled *Best Foot Forward*, is an example of what can be done to reach a large number of practitioners by mail.

The effort began with a vision conceived by a group of child health professionals, parents, and advocates who came together to form the Babies with Special Needs Project (Moore, 1992). The group originally envisioned a CME program, focusing on the primary health care needs of infants and toddlers with chronic illness and disability, to be disseminated in videotape format and accompanied by didactic sessions and printed material. In response to funding barriers, the group had to scale its efforts down. A proposal was submitted to the Department of Education, and Part H funding was secured to develop the newsletter.

An editorial board drawn from the Babies with Special Needs Project oversees the production and content of the newsletter. It was decided that the newsletter would be directed at primary care physicians and would have three sections of content. The first section is titled "From a Parent's Diary" and includes information from a family perspective. The second, titled "Friend of the Family," is authored by a physician and draws from professional experience in treating children with special needs. The third section is an article written jointly by a pediatrician and the state's Part H coordinator and carries the heading "The Part H Companion: A Physician-friendly Guide to Minnesota's Early Intervention System." Copies are disseminated to each member of the Minnesota chapters of the AAP and AAFP as well as other health and education professionals involved in the early intervention system. Distribution reaches more than three thousand individuals.

The partnership between the coalition and the state's AAP and AAFP has been a fruitful one. Continued support from Minnesota's Part H program has allowed for expansion of the newsletter, and a proposal has been submitted to present a two-hour seminar for family physicians and pediatricians at each of four community hospitals.

CONCLUSION

Although different groups have used a variety of formats, themes, and techniques for getting their message across, several commonalities are worth mentioning.

First and foremost, there is the involvement of parents in CME training efforts. Parents have been important partners in the development and implementation of all successful CME efforts of which these authors are aware. This is important on several levels. For one thing, a message is sent every time parents are given the opportunity to share their voices; it acknowledges the fact that parents are the experts. Taking advantage of parents' expertise can also facilitate the planning process relative to CME content. Who else has such intimate knowledge of how the practice of medicine affects families? Who else can tell us how to improve our family-centered skills? In addition, when a parent shares the podium with other professionals, it provides a living example of partnership. This is extremely important for those providers who are used to seeing parents in a "one down" or vulnerable position. Finally, parents can be the most effective motivators of CME efforts. In many ways, they have the most at stake, and their tenacity and perseverance help keep planners and organizers on task and moving forward.

Second, all of the programs mentioned in this chapter have in common an emphasis on collaboration. Much more can be accomplished if groups work together to develop and implement CME programs. Cooperation allows for the pooling of resources, which can, in turn, expedite the planning, logistics, and implementation of programs.

Third, we should note the incremental nature of the process of planning and implementation. Most successful CME efforts have started small and grown with their successes. This allows for piloting strategies and for making necessary changes along the way. Efforts that begin with a small planning group and follow a "grow as you go" strategy seem to fare better than those of groups that plan interminably for a grand-scale operation with one opportunity to succeed or fail. It is also worth noting here that, while collaboration is critical, it is also important to keep the nucleus of people who are involved in the planning small enough to be manageable. Additional reviewers can be invited for comment as the process evolves.

Fourth, CME must be designed to meet people where they live. Physicians should have the opportunity to participate in CMEs in their home community. This is especially important for states with large rural areas far from urban centers. In addition, it is essential to consult representatives from the targeted audience regarding strategies for implementation (dates, time, location, etc.).

Fifth, continuing medical education involves a continuous effort. There is a need for follow-up to CME sessions. All of the program organizers consulted felt that the initial sessions did much to enhance awareness, but that additional material was necessary to reinforce and expand on the original information. Unfortunately, the amount of time for which one can "capture" the average CME audience is very limited. Introductory CMEs can effectively open the discussion about the care of children with special needs, but follow-up must be accomplished to assure early detection and treatment and to continue the dialogue about related issues.

Sixth, the final observation brings us back to the original theme of adaptation. It is necessary to maintain a certain amount of flexibility in program planning so that programs can be tailored to meet the needs of different communities and participants. What works in a large medical center may not fly at a rural community health center, and professionals practicing in different contexts may have very different needs for CME.

In conclusion, it seems that the guiding principle in the development of systems to serve children with special needs is equally applicable to planning CME for the physicians who treat them. The focus should be on providing care that is family centered; efforts should be coordinated between various programs and disciplines; and implementation should be community based to assure accessibility to practitioners.

REFERENCES

American Academy of Pediatrics. (1992). The medical home. *Pediatrics* 90:774.

Brewer, E. J., McPherson, M., Magrab, P., & Hutchins, V. (1989). Family-centered, community-based, coordinated care for children with special health care needs. *Pediatrics* 83:1055–1060.

Green, M., & Haggerty, R. J. (1990). *Ambulatory pediatrics IV*. Philadelphia: W. B. Saunders.

Melmed, R. (1991). A new world order! / Preparing the physicians. *Medical Home Newsletter* 4:2–5.

Moore, J. (1992). Minnesota's *Best Foot Forward*: Looking back, looking ahead. *Medical Home Newsletter* 6:4, 19–20.

Rupert, E. S. (1991). Helping children with special health needs by continuing the education of their doctors! *Medical Home Newsletter* 5:2–8.

Siderits, P., Reiss, J., Span, S., Nackashi, J., & Urbano, T. (1992). Building a partnership for children and families in Florida: Early intervention training for physicians and parents. *Medical Home Newsletter* 7:2, 6–11.

9

Overcoming Obstacles to Early Intervention Referral: The Development of a Video-based Training Model for Community Physicians

Rosalyn Benjamin Darling

> You start thinking in your mind [that something is wrong] as you're examining this child month after month. Here you try to hint. You say, "I'm not really sure. We'll watch it a little longer."
>
> —A pediatrician (in Darling, 1979, p. 207)

> [The neurologist said,] "I think I know what's wrong with your son, but I'm not going to tell you because I don't want to frighten you." . . . We insisted that our doctor refer us to Children's Hospital, but the doctor said, "He's little. Why don't you wait? You don't need to take him there yet." . . . [E]veryone was pablum-feeding us, and we wanted the truth.
>
> —Parent of a child with cerebral palsy (in Darling, 1979, p. 147)

Parents and professionals have often expressed dissatisfaction with the failure of many physicians to diagnose developmental disabilities early in infancy and to make prompt referrals to early intervention programs. Although both parents and children do better when intervention is begun as soon after birth as possible, some pediatricians and other physicians persist in delaying diagnosis and referral. A number of new training programs for medical students and physicians have developed in an attempt to familiarize medical professionals with these disabilities and indications for early referral. Some programs, however, assume a need for diagnosis-based referral, and the time lag between the suspicion of a problem and establishment of a definitive diagnosis can still result in delayed referral for treatment.

Also, some of the newer training programs for practicing physicians require a commitment of several days or longer. Many community physicians consider themselves too busy or they lack interest in an extended training program on developmental disabilities or early intervention. This chapter will present a video-based model that has been successful in increasing physician referrals to early intervention programs. The model is not intended to replace more in-depth training programs (such as those described in chapters 8 and 10) that are being developed nationwide, but rather to supplement these programs and educate, at a single session, large numbers of practicing physicians about the value of early intervention.

REASONS FOR NONREFERRAL

Until recently, future physicians received little training in developmental disabilities. The thrust of medical education was the curing of acute illnesses, which responded to treatment and thus rewarded physicians for their efforts. With the advent of antibiotics, immunizations, and other medical "miracles," however, acute illnesses have become less serious and less prevalent, and many physicians are beginning to recognize the need to turn their attentions to chronic conditions and permanent disabilities, which can be ameliorated but not cured.

As a result of this new interest in developmental problems, a number of training programs have been established for medical students, residents, and practicing physicians. Guralnick, Richardson, and Heiser (1982) developed a curriculum in disabling conditions that was designed as a one-month rotation for pediatric residents, focusing on assessment, diagnosis, attitudes, intervention, and other issues. Similarly, Powers and Healy (1982) reported on a nationwide project to provide a sixteen-hour continuing education program to primary care physicians regarding the child with a disability, the family, the educational system, and the community.

More recently, projects have been developed in a number of states to provide both preservice and continuing education to physicians. Most notably, the Medical Home Project of the Hawaii Medical Association (Peter, 1989, 1992) has developed a comprehensive training course for practicing physicians, which has been replicated in various states. Several projects, such as Parent to Parent of Vermont's Medical Education Project (DiVenere, Frankowski & Stifler, 1991), have implemented courses for medical students and residents based on collaboration between parents and professionals. These and other projects are described in other chapters in this book.

If lack of knowledge were the sole cause of the failure of physicians to make early diagnoses of disabling conditions, such educational projects would surely result in more prompt recognition and treatment of these disorders. No doubt, the proliferation of projects that enhance physicians' awareness of developmental problems will result in earlier referrals to early intervention programs. However, ignorance is not the only reason for failure to diagnose and refer. As the sociological literature has shown, diagnosis is an interactional process that takes place between doctors and patients (see, e.g., Freidson, 1970), and a more complete understanding of the complex dynamics involved in this process is necessary in order to reach out to physicians most effectively.

Studies of physicians have shown that they may delay diagnosis and referral in the case of developmental disabilities for a number of reasons: (1) lack of knowledge; (2) negative socialization; (3) sense of failure; (4) lack of communication skills; (5) paternalism; and (6) uncertainty of prognosis. Each of these reasons will be discussed below. The reader should keep in mind that these conditions do not apply to all physicians. Attitudes and practices regarding developmental disabilities have been changing rapidly in recent years, and many partnerships have been developing among physicians, parents, and early intervention providers.

Lack of Knowledge

As indicated above, ignorance of the facts is at least part of the reason that physicians do not promptly recognize and treat developmental disorders. Until recently, these disorders were not generally included in medical school curricula, and many pediatricians and other physicians left their medical training with little or no direct experience with developmental disabilities or chronic illness. Powers and Rickert (1979) found, for example, that only 27 percent of the practicing pediatricians in their sample thought that medical school and residency training had prepared them adequately to work with children with disabilities. The new programs discussed above should help to facilitate awareness of developmental disabilities in recently trained physicians.

Negative Socialization

Physicians are, first of all, people. As a result, they have been exposed to the same stigmatizing images and negative stereotypes of the disabled as have others in society. As Goffman's (1963) classic study and other studies since have shown, the predominant attitude toward people with disabilities in American society is one of stigma, and those who have been exposed to this attitude tend to regard the disabled with a mixture of fear, suspicion, and discomfiture. Very few physicians have had direct personal experience with children or adults with disabilities.

These comments by a pediatrician in one study illustrate the effects of such negative socialization:

> There are personal hang-ups. You go home and see three beautiful, perfect children; then you see this "dud." You can relate more easily to those with three beautiful, perfect kids. . . . If somebody comes in with a cerebral palsy or a Down's, I'm not comfortable. . . . It's hard to find much happiness in this area. The subject of deformed children is depressing. . . . As far as having a Mongoloid child, I can't come up with anything good it does. There's nothing fun or pleasant. (Darling, 1979, pp. 214–215)

Certainly, societal attitudes toward people with disabilities are changing, and not all physicians hold such negative views; however, those who do are likely to dread having to inform parents of the existence of a disabling condition. No one wants to be the bearer of bad news, and negative socialization predisposes most physicians to regard such news as very bad indeed.

Sense of Failure

The primary focus of medicine is curing, and physicians reap their greatest rewards from successful treatment, which restores normalcy of function. Pediatricians, in particular, are trained to cure the acute illnesses of childhood, and many choose that specialty because they enjoy working with typical nonimpaired children. As one pediatrician said, "Our business is a pleasant business—going into the hospital to see a mother who has just had a [normal] baby" (Darling, 1979, p. 211).

Although permanent disabilities can be ameliorated through treatment, they cannot be cured, causing physicians to feel powerless. As Freidson (1970) has noted, physicians tend to operate within a framework of *professional dominance*, in which *they* control the situation of doctor–patient interaction. Their control is based on their ability to cure. Thus, when incurable conditions are suspected, physicians are sometimes reluctant to give up their positions of power by making a prompt diagnosis. As one pediatrician remarked,

I don't enjoy it. . . . I don't really enjoy a really handicapped child who comes in drooling, can't walk and so forth. . . . Medicine is geared to the perfect human body. Something you can't do anything about challenges the doctor and reminds him of his own inabilities. (Darling, 1979, p. 215)

Lack of Communication Skills

Because they are uncomfortable with their role as bearers of bad news and because of their sense of powerlessness, many physicians delay in making a diagnosis of developmental disability. This delay is reminiscent of similar delays reported in other situations of "bad-news telling," including the diagnosis by physicians of cancer or terminal illness (Clark & LaBeff, 1982; Glaser & Strauss, 1965; Quint, 1965) and law officers' making arrests of accused persons (McClenahen & Lofland, 1976).

Lack of appropriate socialization for the role of bad-news teller and fear of recipients' negative emotional reactions lead to various interactional techniques for avoiding the uncomfortable confrontation. Usually the most commonly noted technique in the situation of diagnosing disability is *stalling*. As Goffman notes, when stalling is employed, "the feelings of the [news recipient] are not brought to a head because he is given no target at which to direct them. . . . [T]here is still a chance that the loss has not really occurred" (1952, p. 458).

Research indicates that four stalling techniques are commonly used by physicians in communicating news of a child's disability to parents: avoidance; hinting; mystification; and passing the buck (Darling, 1979).

Avoidance

In avoidance, the physician denies the existence of a problem, even though the parent may have questioned some aspect of a child's appearance or development.

I asked what was wrong with her ears, and they said not to worry about it. . . . I always thought they told you the truth in the hospital and if you wanted to know anything you should ask. I really thought her ears looked funny and I had this funny feeling, so I asked the doctor, "Is anything wrong?" and he looked right at me and said, "No." (parent of a child with Down syndrome, quoted in Darling, 1979, p. 131)

Svarstad and Lipton (1977) have reported that, in 16 percent of the communications in their sample, professionals denied a diagnosis of mental retardation in informing interviews with parents.

Hinting

In hinting, the physician offers clues to parents and waits for them to verbalize their concerns.

> The first visit I make a note on the chart. Maybe I make a suggestion to the parent by listening longer to the baby's heart or whatever. By the next visit, parents start to ask. With cerebral palsy, I sort of lead them into it. I say, "Wait and see." I hedge. Usually I don't call in specialists for two or three months. It depends on parental pressure. (pediatrician, quoted in Darling, 1979, p. 207)

Mystification

In mystification, the diagnosis is presented in medical jargon or euphemistic terms ("motor delay" or "developmental lag") so that the parent cannot equate it with any known (and presumably dreaded) condition such as cerebral palsy or mental retardation. Svarstad and Lipton (1977) noted that, in 32 percent of the cases in their sample, professionals were vague in conveying a diagnosis of mental retardation to parents. Instead of using the term *retardation*, these professionals employed euphemistic descriptions such as "slow for his age."

Passing the Buck

Because of the availability of specialists, many primary care physicians can avoid making a diagnosis. As one said, "The specialist can slap them with the facts" (Darling, 1979, p. 207). Referral to a specialist, of course, protracts the diagnostic process and may raise parental anxiety.

The need to develop skills for communicating diagnostic information more clearly and directly has been recognized by a number of newer training programs for physicians. Some have used role-playing exercises and feedback through videotaping (see, e.g., Cansler, Sharp & Lorch, 1983) to enable medical students to practice these communication skills.

Paternalism

Haug and Lavin (1981, p. 218) have noted that "the training of physicians lays heavy stress on their taking responsibility for their patients, which would seem to require the authority to be in charge and, if necessary, to take control in order to carry out that responsibility despite patient objections." Many physicians argue that they have a responsibility to protect patients from a truth that they are not ready to hear: "Birth is a traumatic experience. For 24 to 48 hours after birth the mother has not returned to a normal psychological state, so I just say everything is O.K. even if it isn't" (Darling, 1979, p. 205). Freidson (1970, p. 42) argues that the patient is believed to be "too ignorant to be able to comprehend what information he gets and . . . is, in any case, too upset . . . to be able to use the information he does get in a manner that is rational and responsible."

Such paternalism may be based on physicians' sincere convictions or it may be adopted as a rationalization for delaying a potentially threatening confrontation. In either case, it serves to delay diagnosis. In reality, studies have shown (see, e.g., Carr, 1970; Darling, 1979; Dickman & Gordon, 1985; Hewett, 1970; Quine & Pahl, 1986) that parental anxiety is increased rather than alleviated by diagnostic delay and that most parents prefer to be told the truth as soon as possible.

Uncertainty of Prognosis

Many physicians justifiably argue that some infants suspected of having developmental problems turn out to be "perfectly normal." In one study (Holden, 1972), children who appeared to be retarded at eight months of age showed great variability in IQ scores at ages four and seven, leading the author to conclude that mental retardation is not predictable in infancy. Thus, premature diagnosis may be a false alarm that upsets parents unnecessarily. In addition, some disabilities are subtle and in fact difficult to diagnose with certainty until long after a child's infancy. Delaying diagnosis in such cases may be unavoidable.

Diagnostic and prognostic uncertainty, however, are sometimes also used as rationalizations for not informing parents of suspected problems. In a classic study of polio patients, Davis (1960) showed that parents were typically given an overoptimistic outlook by medical personnel who were aware that the prognosis for their children was not good. One treatment staff member said, "We try not to tell them too much. It's better if they find out for themselves in a natural sort of way" (Davis, 1960, p. 44).

Thus, even when physicians are aware of the existence of a developmental problem, they may be hesitant, for a variety of reasons, to inform parents promptly. This delay in diagnosis almost always results in a delay in referral to an appropriate early intervention program. Although some programs only enroll children with a specific disabling condition, many can accept children who are at risk of developing a disability or whose only diagnosis is "developmental delay." Yet, at-risk and delayed children are frequently not referred, because the physician is reluctant to alarm the parents prematurely.

DEVELOPMENT OF THE MODEL

Although educational programs that encourage physicians to diagnose early are certainly needed, most existing programs do not address the problem of diagnostic delay caused by real or functional uncertainty. No amount of educational programming will eliminate diagnostic uncertainty entirely. As I have noted, the causes of this uncertainty are multiple, complex, and, in some cases, unavoidable. Thus, a more pragmatic approach seems to be warranted. In an attempt to increase early referrals to an early intervention program in a tri-county area in Western Pennsylvania, a pilot presentation was developed based on the concept of *referral without diagnosis.*

The presentation was designed for pediatricians and family practice physicians and was included in continuing education programs at two area hospitals and at a meeting of the pediatrics department of one of these hospitals. The presentation used a slide/lecture format and consisted of the following elements: (1) definition of early intervention and a brief overview of the literature demonstrating the efficacy of early intervention programs; (2) discussion of the criteria for referral and the concept of referral without diagnosis; and (3) distribution of brochures listing a number to call for referrals to an early intervention program.

The concept of referral without diagnosis was introduced with quotes from parents that illustrated these facts: most parents are at least vaguely aware of developmental milestones and are suspicious of the existence of a disability before a diagnosis is made; and parents have a need to do something to help their children develop. The fact that early intervention programs provide needed parent support was emphasized. A sample protocol was then presented, illustrating a situation in which an undiagnosed child with a motor delay was referred to an early intervention program. The parent is told that the program "will show you ways to help him learn to sit by himself." Physicians are comfortable with such an explanation, because it is not inordinately threatening to the family.

After the presentations, a number of physicians in the audience informally remarked to the presenter that they were not aware of the possibility of referral without diagnosis and were excited about this option. During the three-year period following the presentations, enrollment in the infant program in the area doubled, and the average age of all children in the program decreased from 30.5 months to 22.05 months; during the last six months of the period, the average age of new referrals to the program was 9.5 months, compared with an average age of 24.35 months for the six-month period just prior to the presentations. Before the presentations, most program referrals (83%) came from secondary sources such as teaching hospitals in the nearest large city, and from various community social service agencies; only 11 percent of the new referrals came from primary care physicians (and the remainder came directly from parents). After the presentations, 46.5 percent of new program referrals came from local primary-care physicians (and 49% from secondary sources).

These results are not based on a controlled study, and factors other than the presentations may have contributed to increasing enrollment and earlier referrals. However, the preliminary findings were encouraging and suggested that physicians are more willing to make referrals for early intervention when they are offered a no-diagnosis option.

The slide/lecture format required the presence of a knowledgeable presenter to show the slides, provide an accompanying narrative, and answer questions. In this form, the presentation could not be easily disseminated. As a result, a video-based presentation was developed, entitled *Early Intervention: The Physician's Role in Referral* (1990). The video, which is forty minutes in length, is designed to be shown during continuing education programs at community hospitals. These programs are generally well attended by area physicians, who need the continuing medical education credits. The model involves the showing of the video and a brief presentation by a local team consisting of a physician, a parent, and an early intervention professional to provide local referral information.

The video was professionally produced and is designed to be "generic," so that it can be used in any state, regardless of eligibility requirements for early intervention. Featured are parents and pediatricians describing their interactions with each other and scenes from a home- and center-based early intervention program, a hospital nursery, and a physician's office. Viewers learn about the value of early intervention for children and their families, including children with and without a medical diagnosis.

In addition to addressing the problem of early referral, the video also shows some of the difficulties faced by parents when physicians do not acknowledge their concerns about their children. Both good and bad examples of parent–physician encounters are described by parents, and one pediatrician acknowledges his discomfort with children with disabilities.

As of this writing the video and accompanying manual, which were produced in 1990, have been requested by and sent (at a nominal cost to cover production and mailing) to more than 150 agencies, libraries, state Part H offices, universities, and individuals in thirty-eight states, two Canadian provinces, and Australia.

The model is also being used in Pennsylvania as part of the state-sponsored Family-Focused Early Intervention System's "Referral Module." Through this statewide technical assistance system, the module will be available to all local interagency coordinating councils for use in community-level physician education.

PRELIMINARY EVALUATION

A questionnaire was sent to all those who received copies of the video and manual before the end of 1992. A total of ninety-five questionnaires was mailed, and thirty-eight (40%) were returned. The unreturned forms can probably be largely explained by two factors. First, for many of the orders, only a purchasing department address was listed; thus, the questionnaire may never have been received by the individual who had actually requested the model package. Second, thirty-five of the packages had been distributed free of charge (through a grant from the Pennsylvania Developmental Disabilities Planning Council) at a Pennsylvania conference, and a number of the attendees probably had no real intention of using the materials.

The thirty-eight responses came from nineteen states and included representatives of various kinds of agencies, as indicated in Table 9–1. As the table shows, the majority of respondents represented early intervention programs or agencies.

Respondents were asked whether they had used the model with a physician or group of physicians or whether they planned to use it in the future. Responses are shown in Table 9–2. As the table shows, 84 percent of the respondents had used or planned to use the model with physicians.

Table 9–1
Affiliations of Respondents to Initial Video Use Questionnaire

Affiliation	Number	Percent*
Early intervention program	20	53%
Parent, or parent group	4	11%
Technical assistance program	3	8%
University training program	3	8%
Hospital-based program	3	8%
Physician, or medical practice	2	5%
Health department, or other community agency	3	8%
Total	38	101%

*Rounded to nearest whole number

Table 9–2
Reported Use and Planned Use of the Model with Physicians

Response	Number	Percent
Have used the model with at least one physician or group of physicians	10	26%
Have not yet used the model but plan to do so:		
within the next 3 months	4	10.5%
within the next 6 months	4	10.5%
within the next year	10	26%
more than a year from now	1	3%
other	3	8%
Total	32	84%
Do not intend to use the model with physicians	6	16%

The six respondents who did not intend to use the model in this way explained that they were using it in other ways, and one noted that their project was ending.

Of those who had already used the model with physicians (ten respondents, including six early intervention professionals, one physician, and three technical assistance specialists), eight (80%) indicated either that physician referrals had already increased or that they expected physician referrals to increase as a result of their use of the model. No one thought that referrals would not increase following use. Two technical assistance specialists did not respond to the question because of the absence of personal experience with the model. A total of ninety-nine physicians was reported to have received training based on the model. Of these, sixty-four were practicing physicians, and thirty-five were physicians-in-training.

Several of the respondents who had used the model made additional comments, including the following:

The staff and I feel that this is a very good video and were pleased that an effective job was done to talk about this subject. For many years we have talked about what you have put on this tape. Thank you!

I am sorry that I cannot be more specific in my answers to your questions. This video is very popular; it is frequently on loan. All feedback has been excellent.

Content is great!

I have 12 hospital NICU's I work at and plan to use this a lot.

Would like a shorter version for use in physician offices.

One interesting, and unanticipated, finding was the extent of the video's use with groups other than physicians. Most of the respondents reported having used it successfully with early intervention staff, special education teachers, parent groups, nurses, local interagency coordinating councils, therapists, service coordinators, multidisciplinary teams, and social workers. One parent (who showed the video to a group of special education teachers) remarked, "[This model] has been sorely needed for years! It will make a difference for families."

Some concern was raised by three respondents (all of them early intervention professionals) who indicated that hospitals or physician groups had not been receptive to their coming to do a presentation. One successful strategy, used by some states, has been distribution of the video and manual through local interagency coordinating councils. Another strategy involves coordination at the state level with the state chapter of the American Academy of Pediatrics. Usually the state chapter has a committee concerned with children with developmental disabilities or special health needs. Members of this committee can be helpful in contacting local physicians.

A further follow-up study is planned for the future, after additional purchasers of the model have had a chance to use it with physicians. These preliminary results are promising, however, and suggest that a one-time presentation to physician audiences can be effective in increasing early intervention referrals.

CONCLUSIONS

As a result of the passage of P.L. 99-457, physician training programs have begun in many places and will probably proliferate in the years ahead. Some of these programs will occur on the medical school and residency levels, and others will involve practicing physicians. The in-depth training that these programs will provide should certainly increase collaboration between physicians and early intervention programs. Until then, however, the video-based model presented here appears valuable as a relatively easy means of reaching a large number of physicians in a short amount of time.

The in-depth analysis of reasons for nonreferral provided in this chapter also suggests that those who are developing physician education models and curricula should become more cognizant of the sociological bases for physician behavior. The field of medical sociology contains a vast literature on physician–patient interaction, and much of that literature is relevant to the situation of communication between physicians and parents of young children with disabilities.

Physicians are, in a way, the gatekeepers of the early intervention system. They are the experts that parents trust to confirm the existence of developmental delays and recommend appropriate treatment. Any successful child-find effort must include outreach to the medical community. This chapter has suggested some reasons for the reluctance of many physicians to make early intervention referrals in the past and has offered a valuable perspective and useful model for increasing collaboration among physicians, parents, and early intervention professionals in the future.

REFERENCES

Cansler, D. P., Sharp, M. C., & Lorch, S. C. (1983, December). *Preparing physicians for interpreting developmental diagnosis*. Paper presented at the HCEEP/DEC Early Childhood Conference, Washington, DC.

Carr, J. (1970). Mongolism—Telling the parents. *Developmental Medicine and Child Neurology* 12:213.

Clark, R. E., & LaBeff, E. E. (1982). Death telling: Managing the delivery of bad news. *Journal of Health and Social Behavior* 23:366–380.

Darling, R. B. (1979). *Families against society: A study of reactions to children with birth defects*. Beverly Hills, CA: Sage.

Davis, F. (1960). Uncertainty in medical prognosis: Clinical and functional. *American Journal of Sociology* 66:41–47.

Dickman, I., & Gordon, S. (1985). *One miracle at a time: How to get help for your disabled child—From the experience of other parents*. New York: Simon & Schuster.

DiVenere, N., Frankowski, B., & Stifler, D. (1991). The medical education project: A shared learning experience—Incorporating principles of family centered care in physician education. *Medical Home Newsletter* 4(2):2, 5–8.

Early intervention: The physician's role in referral. (1990). Video and manual. Johnstown, PA: Beginnings Early Intervention Services of Cambria County.

Freidson, E. (1970). *Professional dominance*. Chicago: Aldine.

Glaser, B. G., & Strauss, A. L. (1965). *Awareness of dying*. Chicago: Aldine.

Goffman, E. (1952). On cooling the mark out: Some aspects of adaptation to failure. *Psychiatry* 15:451–463.

Goffman, E. (1963). *Stigma: Notes on the management of spoiled identity*. Englewood Cliffs, NJ: Prentice-Hall.

Guralnick, M. J., Richardson, H. B., Jr., & Heiser, K. E. (1982). A curriculum in handicapping conditions for pediatric residents. *Exceptional Children* 48:338 346.

Haug, M. R., & Lavin, B. (1981). Practitioner or patient: Who's in charge? *Journal of Health and Social Behavior* 22:212–229.

Hewett, S. (1970). *The family and the handicapped child: A study of cerebral palsied children in their homes*. Chicago: Aldine.

Holden, R. H. (1972). Prediction of mental retardation in infancy. *Mental Retardation* 10:28–30.

McClenahen, L., & Lofland, J. (1976). Bearing bad news: Tactics of the deputy U.S. marshal. *Sociology of Work and Occupations* 3:251–272.

Peter, M. I. (1989). *The pediatrician and the new morbidity, module III: The pediatrician and family centered care*. Honolulu: Hawaii Medical Association.

Peter, M. I. (1992). Combining continuing medical education and systems change to promote physician involvement. *Infants and Young Children* 4:53–62.

Powers, J. T., & Healy, A. (1982). Inservice training for physicians serving handicapped children. *Exceptional Children* 48:332–337.

Powers, J. T., & Rickert, N. (1979). *Physician perceptions of inservice training needs: A working paper*. Evanston, IL: American Academy of Pediatrics.

Quine, L., & Pahl, J. (1986). First diagnosis of severe mental handicap: Characteristics of unsatisfactory encounters between doctors and parents. *Social Science and Medicine* 22:53–62.

Quint, J. C. (1965). Institutionalized practices of information control. *Psychiatry* 28:119–132.

Svarstad, B. L., & Lipton, H. L. (1977). Informing parents about mental retardation: A study of professional communication and parent acceptance. *Social Science and Medicine* 11:645–651.

Waitzkin, H., & Stoeckle, J. D. (1976). Information control and the micropolitics of health care: Summary of an ongoing research project. *Social Science and Medicine* 10:263–276.

10

What Do Physicians Want to Know? A Statewide Survey Report of Physicians' Needs for Information about Early Intervention

Francine Gortler Gallagher
and
Corinne W. Garland

Early intervention services can avert the need for special education when a child reaches school age, minimize the likelihood of institutionalization, and provide support to families (Blackman, Healy & Ruppert, 1992; Seklemian, Scott & Garland, 1993). Early intervention services are defined as educational, health, and social services that support and strengthen the development of very young children who have been identified as developmentally delayed or disabled and their families (Healy, Keese & Smith, 1989). In 1986, Congress acknowledged the importance of and need for a system of early intervention services with the passage of Public Law (P.L.) 99-457, which amended the EHA, or Education of the Handicapped Act (since reauthorized as the Individuals with Disabilities Education Act or IDEA) and included Part H, the Handicapped Infants and Toddlers Program. The program, which was part of a broader piece of legislation affecting children with disabilities, often referred to simply as Part H, provides federal grant monies to states to encourage them to plan and implement a coordinated, comprehensive system of early intervention services. By 1994, each state having participated in the Part H program will have to decide whether that state will provide early intervention services as an entitlement for all eligible children ages birth through two and their families.

The philosophy on which Part H legislation is based requires that early intervention systems be family centered and community based. The law requires interdisciplinary collaboration in order to meet the complex needs of families of young children with disabilities. The active participation of physicians in the interdisciplinary early intervention service system is essential. For physicians to assume their new roles as part of community-based interdisciplinary early intervention teams, they must be familiar with the provisions of Part H legislation, understand the significance of early intervention, and participate in the planning process of statewide systems of early intervention services (Scott & Garland, 1992; Wenger et al., 1989).

The physician is frequently the first of many professionals from whom parents seek advice when they have concerns about their child's development and whom they trust to provide information about their child's development. Physicians' offices are critical entry points to services designed to foster children's medical, social, and intellectual development (Pidcock, 1987; Scott & Garland, 1992; Seklemian, Scott & Garland, 1993). The opportunity for children and families to receive early intervention services is, to a large degree, dependent on physicians who are alert to a wide variety of developmental problems and are aware of where to find services needed by children and families. In a statewide survey of pediatricians by the Virginia Department of Mental Health, Mental Retardation, and Substance Abuse Services (Scott, 1990), an effort was made to identify physicians' continuing medical education needs—the first step toward preparing physicians for their active participation in Virginia's early intervention system.

HISTORICAL PERSPECTIVE

In the early 1950s, the American Board of Pediatrics became concerned with physician training in the area of child development: "It was recognized then that pediatricians had little difficulty answering multiple-choice questions regarding child development yet seemed unable to adapt this didactic knowledge to the clinical management of children with developmental disabilities" (Coury, 1990, p. 52). Leaders in pediatrics advocated for changes in pediatric training. In 1978, the American Academy of Pediatrics (AAP) Task Force on Pediatric Education issued a report describing the problems confronting pediatric education and a list of recommendations to serve as guidelines for pediatric training (Coury,

1990). Recommendations made were based on several statements highlighted in the 1978 Task Force Report: (1) that pediatricians should have the skills to cope with biosocial and developmental problems; (2) that residency programs need to emphasize training physicians to care for children with chronic disabling conditions; and (3) that there is a need to reevaluate and revise reimbursement formulas to encourage pediatricians to manage these roles (Bennett, 1982; Coury, 1990; Scott et al., 1993).

Another landmark effort in pediatric training related to caring for children with disabilities involved the work of the Task Force on Education in Developmental Pediatrics. This task force, coordinated by staff members at the Ohio State University's Nisonger Center, was established in 1978 to develop a curriculum in developmental pediatrics. The curriculum, focusing primarily on children with severe disabilities, was intended for medical residents with fundamental clinical skills, knowledge, and attitudes so that, as practicing pediatricians, they might contribute in the assessment process and in the management of children with disabilities (Blackman, 1991; Coury, 1990; Scott et al., 1993).

Also in 1978, the American Academy of Pediatrics, with funding from the U.S. Department of Education, Office of Special Education and Rehabilitation Services, developed and implemented a continuing education program that reached more than five thousand primary care physicians who serve children with disabilities: "The program was intended to improve physicians' interpersonal and professional attitudes toward children with handicaps, as well as their clinical skills and cognitive language" (Coury, 1990, p. 53). The program developers considered this as "an initial effort in meeting the enormous gaps in training that existed as a result of medical school and residency training deficiencies" (Coury, 1990, p. 53).

In the early 1980s, Project Bridge was developed to provide physicians with training in preparation for their participation as team members on interdisciplinary early intervention teams. Physicians received training in the context of the teams in which they worked, contributing to the success of the training and to their ability to serve as team members (Blackman, 1991; Coury, 1990).

Shonkoff and colleagues (1979) conducted survey research in New England in the late 1970s, revealing that 79 percent of the pediatricians surveyed described their training as inadequate. A national survey conducted in 1979 indicated that 73 percent of the primary care physicians who responded to the survey reported the need for further training to work with children with disabling conditions (Powers & Healy, 1982). In early 1990, a statewide survey of pediatricians by the New York State American

Academy of Pediatrics District II showed that only 15 percent of the participants responded positively to a question asking if they felt well informed about P.L. 99-457 (Blackman, Healy, & Ruppert, 1992; Scott et al., 1993). Very few pediatricians participating in that study responded that they saw themselves as involved in the development of the Individualized Family Service Plan (IFSP)—a written plan for early intervention services for each eligible child and family.

In 1985, Guralnick and colleagues conducted survey research involving all board-certified pediatricians in Ohio (Guralnick et al., 1988). A questionnaire was sent to a sample of 644 pediatricians, with 54.9 percent responding. Guralnick and colleagues examined pediatricians' perceptions of the benefits of early intervention related both to child development and to the family. Overall, pediatricians appeared to view early intervention positively and judged that early intervention produced at least a modest impact on children's development, with the highest impact on children with hearing impairments. Respondents were even more positive about the effect of early intervention for families.

Wenger and colleagues conducted survey research to examine physicians' contributions to state planning for early intervention services and their assessment of the relationship between the private health sector and the public human-services system (Wenger et al., 1989). Of those surveyed, 125 physicians responded, representing an 86 percent response rate. Based on the survey responses, the authors concluded that community-based private physicians should be involved in state-level planning, that states need to develop and support structures for physicians' participation in planning and coordination at the local level, and that states should collaborate with all appropriate state and local agencies and professional organizations.

"A SURVEY OF PEDIATRICIANS ON EARLY IDENTIFICATION AND EARLY INTERVENTION"

Collaborative Effort

The Scott (1990) study, "A Survey of Pediatricians on Early Identification and Early Intervention," was a collaborative effort funded by Part H grant funds through the Virginia Department of Mental Health, Mental Retardation, and Substance Abuse Services. The Director of Child Health, Virginia Department of Health, assisted in the development of the questionnaire used. The 1990 president of the Virginia Chapter of the American Academy of Pediatrics endorsed the study and signed the cover letter.

Research Questions

To obtain information on the current screening techniques, referral practices, and training needs as perceived by the pediatricians in Virginia, the study was designed to answer the following questions:

1. To what extent are pediatricians involved in child-find efforts, including the routine use of developmental screening techniques, and referral of infants and toddlers to local early intervention programs?
2. What are the factors that influence pediatricians to make referrals to early intervention programs?
3. What are pediatricians' perceptions of their educational needs in regard to early intervention service delivery to infants, toddlers, and their families? (Scott, 1990)

Method

Sample

The 965 pediatricians listed in the Virginia Medical Directory of Physicians, published by the Medical Society of Virginia in cooperation with the Virginia State Board of Medicine (1989), were asked to participate in the study (Scott, 1990; Scott et al., 1993). Of those asked, 342 pediatricians responded, yielding a 40.18 percent response rate. Slightly more than half (52.4%) of the respondents were between the ages of twenty-six and forty-five years, and the remainder were forty-six years or older.

The range of participants' dates of graduation from medical school was from 1934 to 1986. Of these, 50 percent of the respondents graduated prior to 1971, and the remainder between 1971 and 1986. When asked about board certification, 297 pediatricians (88.1%) indicated that they were certified by the American Board of Pediatrics. Approximately one-third (32.4%) of the respondents reported formal subspecialty training (e.g., a fellowship in neonatology). Almost three-fourths (74.8%) of the respondents noted that they had received formal training in developmental pediatrics, while eighty-six (25.2%) reported that they had received no such training.

Type of Practice

Approximately two-thirds (66%) of the pediatricians responding were either in a solo practice or a group of two or more physicians, while 18.9 percent identified their practice as being based at a hospital, local health department, or health maintenance organization. When asked about the type of pediatrics included in their practices, 67.6 percent stated general pediatrics only, 14.1 percent indicated specialty pediatrics, and 18.3 percent noted that their practices included both general and specialty pediatrics.

Many of the respondents indicated several of the following choices to show all areas in which they practiced: urban, 23.4 percent; urban/rural, 16.9 percent; regional, 14.5 percent; suburban, 24.3 percent; and rural, 44.4 percent. When asked for the approximate number of infants and toddlers with developmental delays and/or disabilities seen annually by the physician alone (as opposed to the total seen in a group practice), the largest number—51.9 percent—chose the ten-to-fifty category; 32.3 percent indicated the less-than-ten category; and 15.8 percent reported fifty-one or more. Pediatricians participating in the study were also asked to indicate the approximate percentage of infants and toddlers in their practices from home environments they judged to be potentially adverse (e.g., low income; parents with limited education; teenage parents). The majority (64.5%) estimated that 0–25 percent of their patients were from adverse home environments, and almost 20 percent estimated that 26–50 percent of their patients were from adverse home environments.

Instrument

The Pediatricians' Early Intervention Questionnaire was designed specifically for the study. The instrument included five sections presented in the following sequence: (1) background information; (2) developmental screening methods; (3) referral practices; (4) training needs; and (5) demographic information. The questionnaire consisted of thirty-three items with a cover sheet defining the terminology used throughout the survey. Of these items, thirty-two used a checklist format. The number of possible responses varied from two choices per question to checklists of twenty-three choices. One question requested a narrative response regarding recommendations for pediatric residency training programs based on the physicians' personal experiences.

The questionnaire was field tested in Maryland by community-based pediatricians and was modified as a result of the field test. Following the field test, the revised questionnaire was reviewed by a wide range of professionals involved in the planning process for a comprehensive system of early intervention.

Procedures

The questionnaire was mailed to pediatricians with a cover letter signed by the president of the Virginia Chapter of the AAP. A second mailing of the survey, with a reminder notice, was sent seven days after the initial due date to the pediatricians who had not yet returned the survey. Pediatricians serving infants from birth through two years and/or researching services involving infants/toddlers from all regions of Virginia participated in the study. A review of the information available on nonrespondents did not reveal a pattern of nonresponse. The distribution of respondents was fairly equal across five geographic regions of the state.

The data were comparatively analyzed and are presented in a descriptive format using frequency distributions and percentages. Cross tabulations were used to identify significant associations regarding the continuous variables of the year of graduation from medical school, the geographic area covered by practice, and the type of pediatrics included in practice (i.e., general versus specialty).

Results

Developmental Screening Methods

Of the 305 respondents, 97 percent indicated that they screen infants/toddlers routinely as part of well-health supervision. More than half (58.5%) of the respondents reported using standardized screening instruments (e.g., Denver Developmental Screening Test; Prescreening Developmental Questionnaire) regularly during well-child visits. Of these respondents, 82.4 percent of the pediatricians indicated that they were responsible for administering the developmental screening. Other persons cited as responsible for administering the instruments included nurses, nurse practitioners, and health aides. The person administering the screening instrument was trained to do so primarily through a training program. Yet, 65.8 percent of the survey participants identified developmental screening as an area in which they needed continuing education. Most of the pediatricians surveyed (90–94%) indicated screening children at the time of their two-, six-, and twelve-month well-child visits. The second most frequently reported age groups for screening during well-child visits included four, eighteen, and twenty-four months, with percentages ranging from 83–88 percent. Nearly 84 percent of the respondents allowed five to fifteen minutes to administer developmental screenings.

Referral Practices

Physicians were asked what follow-up procedure(s) they used when screening results revealed a deviance or delay in a child's development. More than three-quarters (76.7%) indicated that a referral is made to an appropriate professional—for example, to a speech-language pathologist if the delay noted was in communication development. A referral to an early intervention program (74.4%) was rated the second most frequently used follow-up procedure, and the third highest was a referral for a developmental assessment to an individual or other facility specializing in developmental evaluations (e.g., a child development clinic). When provided with a comprehensive list of eleven conditions for which pediatricians thought early intervention services would be beneficial for the child, the top three ranked items were visual or hearing impairment (95%), congenital abnormalities (93.8%), and environmental risk (89.6%).

Pediatricians were asked to rank up to three reasons why referrals to the local or regional early intervention program were not made. The top three reasons were the following: (1) the pediatricians felt that the programs were inaccessible to families; (2) the pediatricians were unaware of programs in their community; and (3) the pediatricians did not believe that the programs' services would be beneficial to the infants, and they questioned the quality of the services provided. When asked whether or not specialists practiced in the participating pediatrician's office, more than half (56.3%) responded that there were no specialists in their practices.

The final question of the referral section of the questionnaire asked, "When you have made a referral, what types of conditions were present in the infants/toddlers?" Participants were instructed to check all conditions that applied. Infants with hearing and/or visual impairments were noted by 90.6 percent as being referred for services most often. The second most frequently referred group was composed of infants with chromosomal abnormalities, identified by 76.4 percent of the respondents. Infants with a birth weight of less than 1,500 grams were third in frequency of referrals made by the respondents (68.9%).

Continuing Education Needs

Participating physicians were asked to provide written comments regarding their recommendations for pediatric residency training programs, based on their personal experiences. The majority of respondents recommended more training in developmental/behavioral pediatrics. Examples of responses supporting this recommendation were "decrease the time spent in the NICU [Neonatal Intensive Care Unit], increase the time in child psychiatry, development, community clinics and school settings" and "more time in well baby clinic and more familiarity with developmental screening tests." Perhaps the most significant finding related to this question was that the recommendations for more training in developmental/ behavioral pediatrics were made by physicians whose dates of graduation spanned the entire range from 1934 through 1986 (Scott, 1990; Scott et al., 1993).

Developmental screening was the area of continuing education most frequently requested by respondents. It was closely followed by the request for further education regarding public/private community resources in early intervention. The third area of continuing education requested was for an orientation to psychological/educational testing instruments. Pediatricians indicated that they would be most likely to participate in regional continuing medical education seminars.

Frequencies regarding the pediatricians' type of practice were crossed with the number of board-certified respondents. The highest percentage of pediatricians certified by the American Board of Pediatrics represented those who were involved in academics or research or were in the retired/semiretired category. The lowest percentage of the respondents indicated practicing pediatrics in a private practice. The pediatricians' years of graduation were cross-tabulated with the number of pediatricians reporting that they regularly consulted with early intervention programs on a monthly basis. Graduates between 1971 and 1980 yielded the highest percentage (75%) of regular consultation with early intervention programs. The second largest group of pediatricians that reported consulting regularly with early intervention programs was the group that graduated from 1981 through 1990.

To examine the relationship between the ways in which physicians acquired skills in administering screening tests and the training programs in medical schools, the frequencies of methods of acquisition were compared with the year of graduation. Of those surveyed, eighty-seven pediatricians (32%) reported that the skill of administering standardized screening tests was self-taught. Of this group, the highest percentage (52.9%) was shown in the "through 1950" category of graduates. In the 1961–1970 category, only 18.2 percent reported teaching themselves the skill of administering a screening instrument. This correlated with the cross-tabulation illustrating the percentage of pediatricians who acquired the skill through a formal training program such as a residency. Slightly over half (52%) of the "1981–present [1990]" category of graduates learned to administer screening tests through their residency training programs. The similarities of the percentages regarding self-taught pediatricians coupled with the increase in pediatricians learning screening techniques through residency programs indicates that since 1980 more pediatricians are learning to administer screening tests (Scott, 1990; Scott et al., 1993). This finding is encouraging when one compares the results of a 1978 survey revealing that 63 percent of pediatricians responding to a questionnaire ($n = 121$) indicated that they used developmental screening tests, but only 15–20 percent screened more than 10 percent of their patients (Smith, 1978).

A comparison by year of graduation of the pediatricians who requested continuing education in screening techniques revealed that 76.5 percent of the physicians who graduated before 1950 requested more training in this area. The lowest percentage (45.7%) of requests for continuing education in screening techniques was found among graduates from 1971 to 1980. A high percentage of pediatricians (83.2%) noted that they were aware of the provisions of P.L. 99-457, Part H. Of the 83.2 percent, 41.5 percent indicated that they were fully aware of the provisions.

Discussion

A pediatrician's awareness of available community early intervention resources and the timeliness of referrals are the critical factors that influence whether or not children and families receive the services they need. As noted by Shonkoff and colleagues (1979), "optimal care for children with developmental disabilities depends upon maximal utilization of community resources." The survey data indicated that pediatricians were aware of the importance of knowing about community early intervention resources, with 52 percent of the respondents requesting continuing education in this area. As Part H is implemented, "persons and agencies involved in Part H planning must develop ways to ensure that pediatricians are aware of community based early intervention services and perceive them as accessible and beneficial to their patients" (Scott & Garland, 1992, pp. 15–16). The survey data showed a correlation between the kinds of referrals that pediatricians have made and those patients that they thought would benefit from early intervention. For example, 95 percent of the respondents stated that they thought early intervention was beneficial for infants and toddlers with visual and hearing impairments; 90 percent of the pediatricians reported having made referrals for infants and toddlers with visual/hearing impairments. This particular finding also supports findings of a study by Guralnick and colleagues (1988). In this study, the responding pediatricians judged children with hearing impairments to be the most likely to benefit from early intervention. One may conclude that, if pediatricians believe early intervention is beneficial to a child with a certain disability, they will be more likely to refer a child with that type of disability (Scott, 1990; Scott et al., 1993).

The final question posed was, "What are pediatricians' perceptions of their educational needs with regard to early intervention?" More than two hundred pediatricians responded to the open-ended question requesting their recommendations for training, based on their personal experiences. The data clearly suggest that pediatricians recognize a need for more developmental/behavioral pediatrics training to be added to their educational programs in medical school (Scott, 1990; Scott et al., 1993). According to the literature, however, there have been no dramatic changes regarding the content of pediatric training in medical schools (Coury, 1990). In a survey of pediatric practices conducted in New England, 79 percent of the respondents ($n = 97$) rated their formal training in child development as inadequate (Shonkoff et al., 1979). The results of the Scott (1990) study clearly indicate, through a significant number of requests for continuing education dealing with early intervention issues, that physicians need additional information about early intervention in order to assume new roles on community-based teams.

Perhaps the most significant information obtained from the training section of the Scott survey was the extent to which physicians wanted continuing education (Scott, 1990; Scott et al., 1993). Almost two-thirds of the respondents (65.8%) requested more information regarding developmental screening. This indicated not only that pediatricians were willing to learn more in order to participate actively in the identification of infants/toddlers with developmental delays, but also that they identified continuing education regarding developmental screening as a high priority (Scott, 1990; Scott et al., 1993). The three continuing education programs cited as the most likely to be used were regional seminars, local workshops, and annual pediatric chapter meetings devoted to early intervention.

Limitations

There are several limitations to the Scott (1990) study. First, the study was limited to pediatricians in one state, Virginia. However, there is no reason to believe that Virginia pediatricians differ significantly from those in other states or that their responses are in any way atypical of those that would be generated by a national cross-section of practicing pediatricians (Scott, 1990; Scott et al., 1993).

Second, a bias in the sample may have been present in that the pediatricians participating were both interested in early intervention and knowledgeable about the provisions of P.L. 99-457 and also highly trained (Scott, 1990; Scott et al., 1993). Slightly over 80 percent of the respondents indicated their awareness of Part H provisions. In addition, 88 percent of the respondents were certified by the American Board of Pediatrics, exceeding the minimum requirements to practice pediatrics.

Third, another possible limitation of this study is the exclusion of family physicians. Residents in some rural areas in Virginia rely more on family physicians—rather than on pediatricians—for well-child health supervision. However, the range of demographics among those who did respond indicated that the survey elicited a representative sample of physicians serving infants and toddlers across the state (Scott, 1990; Scott et al., 1993).

Implications

The results of the Scott (1990) study have several important implications. The primary implication is that community-based pediatricians must be involved in both planning and implementing Part H at the state and local levels (Scott, 1990; Scott et al., 1993). This finding supports the results of research by Wenger and colleagues (1989) and provides support for the involvement of physicians in early intervention systems (Blackman, 1991; Blackman, Healy & Ruppert, 1992; Coury, 1990; Peter, 1992).

A second implication is the need for additional developmental/behavioral pediatric training in medical school and pediatric residency programs (Scott, 1990; Scott et al., 1993). More than 90 percent of the respondents to the Scott (1990) study recommended that more developmental/behavioral pediatrics training be incorporated into pediatric residency programs. These recommendations were made by pediatricians who graduated from medical school as early as 1934 through as recently as 1986; the need for training was recognized by pediatricians across a wide range of ages and experience (Scott, 1990; Scott et al., 1993). It is important for all professionals involved in early intervention services to be aware of their own roles and those of colleagues from other early intervention disciplines. To promote appropriate referrals and the integration of health and developmental services for infants and toddlers with disabilities, early intervention programs need to ensure that physicians have the information they need to participate actively as team members and to provide physicians with outcome data.

A third implication is the need for continuing education programs for pediatricians in order to promote their active involvement in early intervention services. Continuing education programs provide a mechanism for highlighting the role that physicians are expected to assume, and such programs offer an opportunity for physicians to keep up with new early intervention legislation and methodology. Early intervention personnel are an essential component in the continuing education process for helping to ensure physician participation in community systems of early intervention.

> A majority of the pediatricians in this study [Scott, 1990] indicated that they were aware, although not fully aware, of the provisions of P.L. 99-457. Since early intervention personnel have the latest information on Part H, it is our responsibility to share information with pediatricians, include them in training activities, and educate them on a one-to-one basis. Having information available to physicians could promote their becoming aware of early identification and referral of infants and toddlers at risk for or with developmental delays. (Scott et al., 1993, p. 137)

CARING FOR INFANTS AND TODDLERS WITH DISABILITIES: NEW ROLES FOR PHYSICIANS

Developed, in part, in response to the Scott (1990) survey results, Caring for Infants and Toddlers with Disabilities: New Roles for Physicians (Caring for Infants and Toddlers) is an inservice training project of Williamsburg (Virginia) Area Child Development Resources, Incorporated (CDR). The three-year project is designed to provide continuing education to primary care physicians, thus ensuring that they have the information and skills needed to be full participants in a statewide system of early intervention. Caring for Infants and Toddlers is funded by a grant from the U.S. Department of Education, Office of Special Education Programs, Early Education Program for Children with Disabilities.

Collaborative Effort

CDR staff, physicians at the University of Virginia Medical School, and the Virginia chapters of the American Academy of Pediatrics (AAP), the Pediatric Society of the AAP, and the American Academy of Family Physicians (AAFP) collaborated during the developmental phase of proposal preparation. As a result of coordination and collaboration in project design, the project has strong support from the professional chapters, helping to ensure that it meets both the continuing medical education standards of the medical community and the practical needs of busy community-based physicians.

Training Content

The Caring for Infants and Toddlers project addresses physicians' new roles on community-based early intervention teams engaged in five critical elements of the early intervention system: first, identifying very young children with disabilities; second, making referrals for early intervention services; third, providing developmental evaluations and assessments; fourth, developing and implementing Individualized Family Service Plans (IFSP); and fifth, providing service coordination and delivery (Scott & Garland, 1992; Seklemian, Scott & Garland, 1993). The project provides training based on a set of competencies (see Appendix A) developed by the American Academy of Pediatrics (1988) and adapted by the project. Caring for Infants and Toddlers is based on data reported in the Scott (1990) study indicating that physicians are interested in training that is provided through regional seminars, local workshops, and chapter meetings. The project is designed to make continuing education self-directed to the maximum extent possible, using self-study manuals and accompanying audiotapes as a major portion of the curriculum.

The curriculum includes four levels (see Table 10–1). A 3.5-hour "foundations" course is offered at various times in each perinatal services geographic region. The purpose of the foundations course is to provide an overview of the role of the physician in early intervention. All of the physicians participating in the foundations course receive a self-study manual and four fifteen-minute audiotapes to guide them during the second level, "self-study" and "technical support." A self-assessment of the extent to which they possess the AAP competencies is completed and used to direct their reading in the manual. The second level—the self-study process—is designed to provide a knowledge base in each of four areas addressed by the competencies: (1) child find; (2) evaluation and assessment; (3) IFSP and service coordination; and (4) transition. As physicians work through the self-study program, they are invited to call the project staff (via a toll-free number) with any questions or requests for additional information. Physicians incorporate new knowledge into their family practice during the third level of training, "clinical application." The fourth level, which provides "follow-up" instruction and deals with "communication" skills, is offered at each of the professional academies' statewide annual chapter meetings. Training at the foundations and follow-up levels are done by interdisciplinary teams of project staff, physicians, early intervention program coordinators, and family members.

Nominating Leaders

In an effort to identify physicians who provide exemplary care to children with disabilities, project staff replicated a nomination process first used by Dr. Carl Cooley in New Hampshire (Cooley, 1992). Families and

Table 10–1
Caring for Infants and Toddlers Project, Curriculum Content and Sequence

Level	Format	Duration	Purpose
Foundations	Regional workshops	3.5 hours	To provide an overview of the role of the physician in early intervention.
Self-study & technical support	Manuals/ audiotapes	3 months	To provide a knowledge base in each of four competency areas.
Clinical application	Office practice & community-based intervention teams	3–6 months	To incorporate new knowledge into daily practice.
Communication & follow-up	AAP meeting Virginia	3-hr. workshop	To develop skills in communicating with and supporting families.

Source: Seklemian, Scott & Garland, 1993.

physicians throughout Virginia were invited to nominate primary care physicians who they felt were providing exceptional care to young children with disabilities and their families. More than one hundred nominations were received. From among the group of nominees, twenty physicians were selected to participate in an all-day Statewide Pediatric Leadership Conference—the first requirement for participating as a leader in the project. Selection criteria included the number of nominations received for each physician, the extent to which care was consistent with principles of family-centered care (Shelton, Jeppson & Johnson, 1987), and geographic diversity. Invitations, signed by the Virginia chapters of the AAP (president) and the AAFP (vice-president) and by the project director, were sent to the twenty physicians selected, who were also contacted personally to provide further information for the nomination process, to discuss the level of involvement needed from physicians assuming leadership roles, and to be invited to make a commitment to the project in a leadership capacity. All nominees were recognized by their professional association and by the project staff for having been nominated.

Pediatric Leadership Conference

The leadership conference served as a way of honoring the physicians selected, as the site of a field test for the foundations course, and as preliminary training for physicians to become members of the interdisciplinary teams that would carry out the regional training.

Preliminary data from the leadership training at the conference showed that physicians rated the training as very useful, with a mean score of 4.5 (on a scale of 1–5). The two most frequently cited responses to the open-ended question asking "What information presented will be the most useful to you?" were hearing the parents' perspectives that were shared during the panel discussion and receiving the self-study manual as a resource (Seklemian, Scott & Garland, 1993).

Project Evaluation

To measure the effectiveness of all Caring for Infants and Toddlers project activities, and to show that the model of inservice training is replicable, the evaluation participants include project staff, consultants, participating physicians, community-based early intervention providers, and families participating in early intervention (Seklemian, Scott & Garland, 1993). The evaluation plan includes field testing of the foundations-level workshop and curriculum materials prior to regional training, participant evaluation of all training and curricular materials, physician pre/posttest of curriculum content, measure of physician perception of role, measure of infant-program-provider perception of the role of the physician, and measure of family perception of the role of the physician.

Project Significance

Several implications for further research, for systems planning, and for continuing education arise from the original Scott (1990) study and from the initial activities of the Caring for Infants and Toddlers project. It is clear that the state chapters of the AAP and AAFP constitute a powerful and influential organizational structure through which physicians can be reached both for researching their role in early intervention and for encouraging their participation in statewide systems of early intervention. Further, an active role by the professional academies in planning and conducting continuing medical education programs ensures that those programs respond to their constituencies' needs and gives continuing education programs the credibility necessary to attract busy physicians who must choose their continuing education carefully.

While the results of the Scott (1990) survey pointed to the needs of physicians for training in content related to Part H of IDEA, and while several models—including Caring for Infants and Toddlers—have addressed those needs in part, there is still a great deal to be learned about how to plan and deliver continuing medical education that will increase both the amount and the value of physician participation in community systems of early intervention. The Scott (1990) study offers some clues as to the time and place for such training—which influenced the Caring for Infants and Toddlers plan for offering regional training as well as workshops at the annual academy meetings. Caring for Infants and Toddlers offers training in each of Virginia's seven perinatal regions—at different times and locations within each region—to enhance accessibility. The extent to which these strategies, and the use of manuals and audiotapes for self-directed study, will be successful have yet to be measured.

As we examine the content and methodology of Caring for Infants and Toddlers and other continuing medical education models designed to enhance physician participation in community-based early intervention, there is uncertainty as to whether these curricula will, in fact, result in an increase in the quality of care that families value, as indicated in their exemplary-physician nominations. While initial project data—based on the leadership-training evaluation results—suggest that the project can succeed in increasing knowledge and competencies regarding the mechanics of identification and referral (i.e., child find), assessment, IFSP planning, and transition, a great deal remains to be learned about whether or not this project and others like it are successful in helping physicians and other professionals on the early intervention team to carry out their roles in ways that are most supportive to families.

REFERENCES

American Academy of Pediatrics. (1988, November). *Proceedings from a National Conference on Public Law 99-457: Physician Participation in the Implementation of the Law.* Washington, DC: American Academy of Pediatrics.

Bennett, F. (1982). The pediatrician and the interdisciplinary process. *Exceptional Children* 48:306–315.

Blackman, J. A. (1991, June). Why physicians are (or are not) enthusiastic about early intervention. *Early Childhood Reporter* (LRP Productions, Alexandria, VA).

Blackman, J. A., Healy, A., & Ruppert, E. (1992). Participation by pediatricians in early intervention: Impetus from Public Law 99-457. *Pediatrics* 89:98–102.

Cooley, W. C. (1992, June). On golden pond. *Medical Home Newsletter*, pp. 2, 9–10.

Coury, D. L. (1990). Training physicians for increased involvement with children with special needs. *Infants and Young Children* 2:51–57.

Guralnick, M. J., Heiser, K. E., Eaton, A. P., Bennett, F. C., Richardson, H. B., & Groom,

J. M. (1988). Pediatricians' perceptions of the effectiveness of early intervention on at-risk and handicapped children. *Developmental and Behavioral Pediatrics* 9:12–18.

Healy, A., Keese, P. D., & Smith, B. S. (1989). *Early services for children with special needs: Transactions for family support*, 2nd ed. Baltimore: Paul H. Brookes Publishing.

Peter, M. (1992). Combining continuing medical education and systems change to promote physician involvement. *Infants and Young Children* 4:53–62.

Pidcock, F. S. (1987). Developmental screening techniques for pediatricians. *Pediatric Basics* 47:7–11.

Powers, J. T., & Healy, A. (1982). Inservice training for physicians serving handicapped children. *Exceptional Children* 48:332–346.

Scott, F. (1990). *A statewide survey of pediatricians on early identification and early intervention*. Richmond: Virginia Department of Mental Health, Mental Retardation, and Substance Abuse Services, Part H Office.

Scott, F., & Garland, C. W. (1992, March). Assessing and remediating pediatricians' needs in early intervention. *Early Childhood Reporter* (LRP Productions, Alexandria, VA).

Scott, F. G., Lingaraju, S., Kilgo, J. L., Kregel, J., & Lazzari, A. (1993). A survey of pediatricians on early identification and early intervention services. *Journal of Early Intervention* 17:129–138.

Seklemian, P., Scott, F., & Garland, C. (1993). *Caring for infants and toddlers with disabilities: A self-study manual for physicians*. Lightfoot, VA: Child Development Resources.

Shelton, T. L., Jeppson, E. S., & Johnson, B. H. (1987). *Family-centered care for children with special health care needs*, 2nd ed. Washington, DC: Association for the Care of Children's Health.

Shonkoff, J., Dworkin, P., Leviton, A., & Levine, M. (1979). Primary care approaches to developmental disabilities. *Pediatrics* 64:506–514.

Smith, R. D. (1978). The use of developmental screening tests by primary-care pediatricians. *Journal of Pediatrics* 93:524–527.

Wenger, M., McLauren, J., Guild, P., Loda, F., Gallagher, J., De Friese, G., Rich, L., & Bergsten, C. (1989). *Physician involvement in planning for P.L. 99-457 Part H: Interagency coordinating council roles and systems planning issues*. Chapel Hill, NC: Carolina Institute for Child and Family Policy.

APPENDIX A: CARING FOR INFANTS AND TODDLERS WITH DISABILITIES— NEW ROLES FOR PHYSICIANS (Competencies on Which Curriculum Is Based)

Child Find

The primary care physician will:

1. display an awareness of the importance of developmental and family issues.
2. know the components and intent of P.L. 99-457 and the policies and

procedures of their state relative to screening, identification, and referral of children to Part H services.

3. know the criteria for eligibility within their state for Part H services.
4. be able to identify factors placing a child at-risk for developmental delay with particular emphasis on those factors making a child eligible for Part H services.
5. have and regularly employ strategies in a variety of settings (e.g., newborn nursery, hospital stays, well-child office visits) for the observation and identification of children who have disabilities, developmental delays, or who may be at-risk for delay.
6. be skilled in the use and interpretation of developmental screening techniques.
7. have a strategy for providing periodic screening in the context of office-based primary care including:
   a. developmental screening of all infants;
   b. periodic rescreening for all children.
8. know and use the procedures for referring infants and toddlers to the Part H services within the community, and know the variety of community resources available for infants and toddlers who may be eligible.
9. have and regularly use a variety of strategies to enhance linkages and coordination of care including making and receiving referrals to and from secondary and tertiary care settings, risk registries, and other relevant consultants.
10. have and regularly use a variety of strategies for increasing family awareness of developmental milestones, resources for assessment, the importance of early identification, potential for improved outcomes, etc.
11. have and regularly use a variety of formal and informal interview techniques to elicit family concerns and observation regarding the development of their infants and toddlers.
12. have and use communication skills and strategies appropriate for ensuring family understanding of medical information, including consultant findings, and for ensuring their involvement in decisions about referral to Part H or further evaluation and intervention.
13. have strategies and routines for the acquisition of new state of the art knowledge base related to this area.

Assessment

The primary care physician will:

1. be aware of options for his/her own involvement in assessment, diagnosis, and management of the child's health needs based on interests and skills,

and be able to communicate clearly that degree of involvement to parents or caregivers.

2. be skilled in interpreting diagnostic information and implications of diagnosis with family, including eliciting their ideas and concerns.
3. know and use resources for obtaining consultation from other Part H providers when necessary and be skilled in presenting need and rationale for consultation to family.
4. be able to interpret all findings for the family in an understandable way and involve and support family in decisions related to additional assessment, referral, and intervention.
5. be able to perform longitudinal monitoring of a child to clarify trends of growth or function, when appropriate.
6. be able to provide family with options for referral and to make appropriate referrals to agencies providing needed services.
7. be able to present information related to the child's medical condition and functional level to family and other team members responsible for development of a plan of intervention.
8. be skilled in formal and informal interview techniques to allow families to share their strengths and needs related to their child's development and provide emotional support in the process.
9. be skilled in formal and informal interview techniques that encourage families to share their own perceptions of their child's problems, strengths, and needs, and that help families clarify those perceptions.
10. be aware of community resources and have skills in helping families obtain the services they desire.

Developing and Implementing IFSPs

The primary care physician will:

1. be aware of P.L. 99-457 and of principles of family-centered intervention plans.
2. be able to define and arrange medical consultations required for the child's assessment, diagnosis, and ongoing management in a manner consistent with the self-selected degree of involvement and to maintain communication with consultant.
3. know and be able to discuss with a family the value of an IFSP, and know how to initiate or help a family initiate a group process to begin IFSP development.
4. assist family in determining who should be involved in the IFSP process.

5. know the procedure for referral to local early intervention service provider(s) responsible for IFSP development and help family in arranging for their participation.
6. be able to communicate, as a member of the IFSP team, the child's medical and health needs either directly or through the parent to the team.
7. be able to help other members of the IFSP team understand the impact of those conditions on a child's overall development and implications of medical conditions for program planning.
8. assist the family in preparing for the IFSP development, providing support throughout the process, and encouraging the family to be heard and have a principal role in the IFSP development.
9. present and clarify information gained during assessment about the child's conditions, functional levels, family strengths and needs, in sufficient detail to be useful in the IFSP.
10. be able to function as the coordinator or liaison regarding child's health or medical needs, communicating with the child's case manager or other person representing the team providing early intervention services.

Transition

The primary care physician will:

1. understand the stress associated with transition from one service to another for the child and for the family.
2. be aware of community-based early intervention systems that may provide services for children leaving the hospital and returning home (see competencies related to child find and referral).
3. be aware of the criteria which might lead to the termination of early intervention services and help the family become aware of the possibility of discharge from early intervention.
4. be aware of other services for children leaving early intervention programs and be able to provide information about services to families.
5. know how to make a referral to public schools for preschool special education services and know the criteria for eligibility.
6. know the advantages of integrated placements for children with disabilities, be aware of options for integrated placements, and be able to communicate that information to families.
7. participate as a member of the team in developing plans for transition to be incorporated in the IFSP.
8. have communication skills needed to encourage and support families in developing plans for transition to be incorporated in the IFSP.

9. have communication skills needed to encourage and support families and children during the transition to services after early intervention.
10. be aware of the need for and value of service coordination after early intervention.
11. know other resources for service coordination in the community and provide that information to families.

Part III

Directions in Medical Education and Family-centered Care: Prospects for the 1990s and Beyond

11

Health Care for Children with Disabilities: A Contemporary View

Alfred Healy

This chapter is a transcription of Dr. Healy's general session address at the conference "Creating Family–Professional Partnerships: Educating Physicians and Other Health Professionals to Care for Children with Chronic and Disabling Conditions," Pittsburgh, Pennsylvania, May 21–22, 1992.

In my view of contemporary health care for children with disabilities, there are only three factors in the equation that we need to consistently deal with: the child, the family, and the community of resources that are available to support and nurture that child and family. You can slice it and dice it or repackage it, rename it, reconfigure it, but the equation always contains those three factors: the child, the family, and that broad community of resources that are available to assist the child and family.

I like to show this particular slide of Sherri and her mother. In one way it does bring together that equation. There's a child, part of a family, standing in front of a resource that's available to them in the State of Iowa: the University Hospital School. But it's not the real reason I want to show this particular shot. The real reason is the joy on the face of that mother, who totally enjoys her child who also happens to have a significant problem with a myelodysplastic lesion. Sherri has ambulatory problems, has some mild to moderate cognitive problems, certainly has bowel and bladder problems. Yet, Sherri's mother is absolutely pleased with her. The attitude that this mother has, and that the entire family has, in not "accepting" but coping and dealing with Sherri's problem is really why we are here today and what this is all about: bringing together people who have the appropriate attitudes, who can assist Sherri and her mother to make total use of what they have through the resources available to them.

I will keep coming back to the issue of attitude. This poster from the Association for Retarded Children puts a finger on it: "My problem isn't how I look; it's how you see me." How we as professionals communicate that—both verbally and nonverbally—and how we approach problems will suggest and strongly communicate our attitudes and values regarding children with disabilities and their families.

Those three factors of child, family, and community interrelate. On a daily basis we must identify the strengths and needs of that child and family, and match those needs with the resources available in the larger community. We must identify, evaluate, plan, implement, and modify as we meet those needs. My major premise here this morning is that, until we have some common principles on which we build that process of identifying, evaluating, and planning, we will often go astray as we make administrative and regulatory decisions. We've got to have basic principles that guide our decisions. Principles should be generic to both provider and consumer. You cannot write different principles for either side of that equation; they must match. Once you have principles identified, you can communicate directly with parents, family members, health care providers. Five years ago, we developed just such principles in four publications through a grant from the U.S. Bureau of Maternal and Child Health. We wrote *Guidelines for Physicians*, *Guidelines for Families*, *Guidelines for Therapists*, and *Guidelines for Social Workers*. They all use the same generic principles of health care, but they're expressed in terms which will assist in operationalizing them within the different disciplines. The principles remain the same. They cannot vary—or you risk having a system that includes inequities. The basic principles should be broadly interdisciplinary. They must apply to physicians, social workers, nurses, therapists, audiologists, and nutritionists. Although the way these principles are operationalized may vary between disciplines, no one has the right to violate the principles of others or to have their own special principles of care.

Qualitative aspects of the basic principles should be applicable in all settings. I'll speak to this using the health care system as an example. The health care system has divided itself into three tiers or levels of service: primary, secondary, and tertiary. One of the major mistakes that's made when we start talking about those three levels is to do so in a way that implies a difference in quality between the services provided. The only difference is in the array of services available to the child and family. The quality should be the same. Primary care should be of the same high quality as the most expensive and comprehensive care available in a tertiary university-based setting. So, basic principles should be applicable in all settings, across the board.

What are those principles? After much discussion with a wide variety of individuals, we organized them into four broad areas. We must,

1. Assure access to quality services.
2. Focus on the child and family unit.
3. Support normal living patterns in the home and community.
4. Promote better health care for children in the future.

Let's look at the first one, which involves assuring access to quality services. What are we talking about? As most of you are aware, the access issue includes fiscal and other barriers to care. Assuring access means providing the best medical knowledge and treatment available. We have interviewed several hundred families, including some from Ireland; and every interview confirms parents' desire that this principle be in place and inviolate. They want to be sure that the best medical information, knowledge, and treatment is available to them. According to our families, all other issues of service delivery paled in comparison, even when we included financing. Assuring access means that we must move to deliver a comprehensive range of health, education, and social services. Obviously, this gets into political and fiscal considerations. However, if you do not build a system based on principles, this concept of comprehensiveness is very easily violated.

Fostering coordination and communication between the child and family with all service providers is a part of assuring access. The spirit of cooperation and collaboration needs to be extended into all of our interactions.

The second principle is that focus must be on the child and family unit. Although these principles were developed earlier, this is reminiscent of the Surgeon General's banner of family-centered, community-based, comprehensive, coordinated care. It means recognizing parents and children as active participants in the decision-making process. I don't mean in a perfunctory manner; I mean full participation in those decisions.

We must assist the child and family to become informed and knowledgeable about health care services. This doesn't mean that we expect them to know how to get that kind of information, but that we actively assist them in obtaining it. This means that we must also work toward solving those problems of time and compensation involved in getting adequate information. Right now there's no way that can be compensated within the health care field. We've got to work on getting the process to respect that principle.

Focusing on the child and family unit also means respecting religious values, cultural diversity, and financial integrity of the family unit. This last piece—respecting the financial integrity of the family—can be especially difficult when legislators and other fiscal intermediaries are making decisions totally based on fiscal implications, without regard for the actual needs of the child. All three, however, are important in helping the child to attain the highest level of achievement at home, school, and within the community.

The third principle is to support normal living patterns in the home and community. This refers to the effort to recommend treatment options that are least disruptive for families in terms of time, expense, and coordination of services. It may mean working against the orthopedic surgeon who says, "We've got to do these hips tomorrow"—which will disrupt the child's educational experience for six weeks to two months, to do a procedure that can wait to be scheduled at a time that will not disrupt the child's full participation in family, school, and community activities. We must be vigilant about this principle because it is one that is too often violated.

By its nature, this third principle means promoting the use of services close to home. This can be tricky, because absolutely all services that a child might need are not necessarily found in the community. I believe that this principle requires that a broad array of primary and secondary services must be available in communities, but that we must balance this with fiscal responsibility. As a nation, it may not be fiscally possible to have tertiary facilities with broad comprehensive programs in every community. There may be some travel required to get to the more complex services. We do need to be continually assessing how far we should expect parents to travel in order to get these complex services. However, the basic principle remains the same, and we must encourage the development of those services that are unavailable and fiscally appropriate.

And [the] fourth [principle is to] promote better health care for children in the future. What we're doing today is building for tomorrow. This means we must work on individual and systems change. Every action that we are taking in the name of an individual child has long-term implications. These must be at least contemplated and thought through. We don't know all the answers. We certainly know a lot more than we did twenty years ago, but we have a considerable way to go until we understand it all. Therefore, each one of us must take an advocacy role to change the system so that, in the future, individual children will have a better shot.

The next step after formulating the basic principles is to operationalize them. How do we do it? We can implement these with a five-step process. This is nothing new; you know all of this. First you establish a collaborative relationship with some part of the system or a provider. You then identify problems of the strengths and needs of the child. This means that you include the areas of health, cognitive, social, and psychosocial functioning. You have to look at a broad array of functions. Step three is to develop an individual plan of care based on the identified strengths and needs of the family and child. Step four involves follow-up to promote the needed care. We often fail at this point because we fail to indicate a time frame and some objectivity to the expected results. Clearly outlined objectives are necessary to facilitate constant monitoring and evaluation of what's going on. The fifth step is to participate in outreach and advocacy activities. This is, then, a five-step process that puts in place those four principles.

I might just mention here that, as I talk here, I am using "children" to include infants, children, and adolescents. When their participation is suggested, we intend it to be within the limit of their abilities. "Parents" is used as a generic term to include all of the nurturing social units, whether they be single parents or the more traditional family units, adoptive parents, fostering parents, or whatever the situation may be.

Physicians must be made partners in the process. I firmly believe in this. [First,] it's important to remember that professionals must understand the system in which they are expected to work. You cannot ask physicians to work in early intervention unless they understand what early intervention is all about. Secondly, they must understand the role that we expect them to play in that system. They've got to know exactly what their role is, relative to others in the system. Third, they've got to possess the knowledge, skills, and attitudes to play out those roles. And fourthly, you've got to pay them to do it—in the same way as every one of us in this room likes to be compensated for what we do. We must remember that the physician and the parent are traditionally the only ones in IFSP [Individualized Family Service Plan] and IEP [Individualized Education Program] meetings that are expected to be there without compensation. Or if they expect it, they're very seldom compensated within the system that we have at the present time. So, in addition to the issue of time constraints, that of compensation also becomes critical. We must remember that the time physicians spend in uncompensated activities is also time away from activities that he or she would otherwise be compensated for. So, if you want to increase physician participation in early intervention, or any other school-based programs or chronic-health-care programs, keep these four basic principles in mind.

As an example of the kinds of attitude changes we need to instill, I'd like to share with you a statement directly out of a 1973 Smith and Wilson's textbook: "Every baby with or without Down syndrome is a unique person. The child with Down syndrome, like other children, has a potential, but it's a limited one." In many, many ways, Smith and Wilson is an excellent text. It was one of the first that really addressed the need to educate parents about their child with Down syndrome. But that statement—is that basically a true statement? Possibly. But does it embody the attitude that we want physicians, therapists, educators, and nurses to evince as they apply their knowledge? No, I don't think so. It's exactly the same as if we approached every junior medical student and taught them that leukemia is a fatal disease. To a certain extent this is true: Leukemia is a fatal disease. However, with treatment, 80 percent of individuals with leukemia lead full, productive lives. If we don't teach the total message, we are doing a disservice to those whom we are responsible to educate. They need to intellectually understand the first part, but operationally, the second part must be brought into play.

I'd like to spend some time now reviewing what needs to be in place in a comprehensive system of care if we respect those four basic principles. It starts with, as far as we're concerned, an appropriate family life education for every student, kindergarten through twelfth grade. Call it anything you want: Life education, growth and development, life skills—whatever it is, it's informing children from the very earliest age about the facts of life. This includes their potential for parenting, the need to be involved citizens at all levels, and some basic facts about parenting children, including children with chronic illness or disabilities. This is so that, as they approach parenthood—the only job in life which we ask of them for which we present no education—they might be in a position to become positively involved.

Preconceptional counseling should be available for every couple contemplating parenthood. This means we would have the means to assist potential parents in understanding the risks and responsibilities of parenthood and to make them knowledgeable partners in wanting children. Many are now speaking to this point, nationally. We are going to hear far more in the future about the logical sequence of wanting a child, participation in prenatal care because you want that child, and the resultant reduction in prematurity—which reduces the single factor most causally related to disabilities. You will have wanted children, you will increase participation in prenatal care, you will reduce prematurity, and you will reduce the incidence of disabilities. This equation has considerable significance.

Genetic counseling services must be available at appropriate times. Keep in mind that I'm separating genetic from preconceptional counseling. Genetics is a part of it, but preconceptional counseling has a far broader approach to the assistance of potential parents to want and nurture children.

In addition, there is growing awareness of the importance of optimal prenatal counseling and associated services. An appropriate level of obstetrical and perinatal care must also be available if we are to minimize risk. The most optimal transportational vehicle, if you will, for an at-risk infant is still the womb. This means that a child has a better chance at a positive outcome if high-risk pregnancies are identified early and referred to a center where appropriate perinatal care is available.

Early and accurate identification of the needs of newborns, with referral to appropriate service systems, is essential. This is where the pediatrician comes in. Every pediatrician is interested in certain aspects of pediatric care. I became interested in children with disabilities and long ago left behind the idea that I might want to be a surgeon. I have no interest in surgical care. No one is forcing me to be a surgeon, but yet no one forced me to be interested in developmental care. I spontaneously and personally chose that part of pediatrics. But there are others who do not necessarily enjoy or derive satisfaction from working intensively with children with disabilities. I think we need to respect that. However, there are some basic aspects of pediatric care that relate to children with disabilities. Let me illustrate this with an analogy. A mother brings a child with what appears to be appendicitis to see a pediatrician. The pediatrician says, "Yes, that is appendicitis. Here's the Yellow Pages. Find a surgeon." That's not very appropriate contemporary care. Appropriate contemporary care requires that pediatricians, the moment they set up practice, need to find and select appropriate surgical colleagues to whom they may refer the cases they do not feel comfortable with or have the skills to deal with. I think a similar responsibility exists for the pediatrician or the family physician who is not personally interested in the care of children with disabilities. They need to have a referral process in place so that, the moment they see a child who either has or shows early signs of a disability, they can get that child to a physician who does have an interest in those kinds of children and families. This does not mean a high-priced, high-level consultant, but rather a pediatrician who will meet the needs of that child and family. This is their basic responsibility; they can't just shrug it off and say, "Well, that's not my bag, that's not my cup of tea." They would not hand the Yellow Pages to a child in need of surgical services; but, in essence, that's what is done too often in pediatric offices, for children who need services related to disabilities.

This process should include a mechanism for identification of those at biological or environmental risk who may be in need of services at a later date. Pediatricians and family practitioners must put together some type of a high-risk follow-up process. This means that services need to be in place for these families. It's expensive and it's difficult, especially for children at environmental risk; but if we are to have comprehensive systems of services, this needs to be looked at. We are having significant problems in this area. Why do I say that? Eighty percent of the children who eventually end up in special education are unknown to the system at two years of age. This means that the process of early identification of high-risk children needs to be strengthened.

In the realm of service delivery, we need evaluation and diagnostic services to specify the needs and strengths of individuals and families, communication and referral systems to ensure that needs are matched with appropriate early intervention services, and well-conceived home- and center-based early intervention services responsive to specific individual and child needs. The availability of early intervention services is improving. Turfism or models of special education that are watered down for infants and young children are decreasing. I think the message is finally getting out that early-childhood special education is different. It requires different preparation; to a large extent, it requires different personnel and it requires different curricula. We are increasingly recognizing that it is a different system. We also need total and complete acknowledgment of the right of the family to be intimately involved. In addition, we need methods to track, monitor, and revise early intervention services.

The process of transitioning to and from "special" systems of care needs to be part of the system. Early and comprehensive communication between those guiding the child either to transition to special education or assisting the child and family to exit the service system is essential. This is traditionally considered a problem in the transition following early intervention. Right now, one of the single greatest needs in our health care system for children with disabilities is the need to transition children from special education into the adult system. That transition is one area where we have failed miserably. Those of us in academia have considered the problem at length; however, in practice there is often nowhere for children with disabilities to transition to for health care. Family physicians aren't interested; internists are not interested. The only solution that we have identified so far is for continuing care provided by pediatricians. This is less than optimal. This is a major issue that all of us concerned with health care issues for children with disabilities and chronic illness must face.

Let us turn now to the issue of what are the competencies that are required by physicians. This was addressed at a conference about two years ago and published in a monograph entitled *Proceedings from a National Conference on Public Law 99-457—Physician Participation in the Implementation of the Law*. This can be secured through the American Academy of Pediatrics. We basically outlined three areas where physicians need to be intimately involved: child find; child assessment; and developing and managing an individual family service plan. (The IFSP is specified because the program was specifically oriented to P.L. 99-457.)

In these three arenas, individual physicians have responsibilities on two levels of care: one at the clinical level in relationship to each and every patient they see; and the second on a systemic level. This means that they have a responsibility—within their individual community, within their state, and, if they have the particular disposition to work at a national level, to see that systems are appropriately put in place. This implies not just a responsibility to an individual child, but to the system of care itself. The Academy has gone on record as saying that that is appropriate and strongly recommended.

I wanted to talk a little bit, before I conclude, about the whole concept of prevention. It is "the play of the future." There are two broad areas to be considered. Number one is the concept of self-advocacy. Where the 1980s brought an emphasis on family care, the 1990s will bring an emphasis on self-advocacy. This means that we are going to need to teach persons—right from their earliest elementary years—how to advocate for themselves, how to represent themselves, and not just rely upon families and other advocacy groups but how to advocate in their own right.

The second broad issue of the 1990s is going to be prevention of disabilities. The National Institute of Medicine and a variety of other groups have come out with a very nice graphic. It basically indicates that there are factors which come together to cause incidents in our lives, which are played out through pathology, impairment, and functional limitation, which can end up in a disability affecting the quality of a person's life. The top of that graphic reflects the interrelationship between biology, environment, lifestyle, and behavior. Up until now, the influence of lifestyle has been played down. I think it's an important addition to the equation, especially when individuals can make choices about their lifestyle. Some elect to continue living in high-risk situations when they do not need to. Smoking, obesity, and avoidance of cancer detection—all three of those factors interrelate to provide some type of an incident or an event in a person's life that relates to pathology.

Let me illustrate this with an example of a child who, as a result of a variety of biologic and environmental circumstances, had an intraventricular bleed in the neonatal nursery. The event was the bleed; the pathology, then, was the brain lesion: a paraventricular leukomalacia. That pathology then led to a malfunction within the cortical spinal tract, which caused the impairment: loss of control over muscles. This resulted in a functional limitation: The child then could not use those muscles, later on, in order to ambulate or manipulate objects. The disability was his inability to participate in a variety of life activities—which then affected his quality of life. That whole sequence is being examined in a variety of ways. For example, we are considering how those risk factors interrelate in ways that produce the incidents or events that produce pathology that leads to functional impairment. We also examine how that functional impairment impacts the quality of life for our children.

The flip side of that whole sequence is this: every complication, as far as I'm concerned, relating to the population that we're dealing with is definable, understandable, and, in many instances, preventable. We know the sequence of complications that occur in a child with spina bifida. We know the sequence of occurrence of complications in the life of a child with cerebral palsy or mental retardation. You can sit down and predict what those complications will be in a gross sense. In the vast majority of instances, they are preventable. For example, I had no concerns regarding scoliosis for the first child I ever treated with spina bifida, because I had never seen a patient that had lived longer than ten years with spina bifida. Now we know that spina bifida—because of the neuromuscular skeletal events—causes scoliosis. We start day one trying to prevent scoliosis. There's a considerable fiscal savings, there's a considerable family and child energy savings, if you attend to those aspects of the child's life that you know can be prevented. Similarly, we can prevent a host of problems by considering appropriate positioning for children with cerebral palsy. It's well known that, if you don't appropriately position the head and neck, complications occur. So the prevention of secondary complications is going to be, then, another major concern of the '90s.

Yet, as I say that, I realize that we must extend our questioning to ask, "What are we creating that we yet don't know about?" What problems are we going to look back upon twenty years from now and say, "Holy cow, how could we have been so stupid?!" We must learn to anticipate the problems which may be created by our interventions. That's what concerns me, and, I think, what has to concern us all. Thirty years ago I actively counseled parents of children with Down syndrome to institutionalize their child, because that was contemporary. That was what I was taught to do. That was the thing to do. One of the greatest experiences of my life has been the relationship I've had with the first parents whom I encouraged to keep a child with Down syndrome. It just so happens that the family are essentially neighbors of mine. I see the child almost weekly, and I see the very positive results of the decision his parents made long ago. He is a fully functioning young man, integrated both into his family and into the community. It's been a very reinforcing sight for me over the years. So I ask you, as professionals involved, to examine what you are doing right now that's supposedly contemporary which might lead us—twenty years from now—to say, "Wow, did we miss the boat!"

I'm a firm advocate of giving kids control of their lives environmentally. Give them the power to move about and to make their own decisions regarding how they want to participate. I think that's the appropriate thing to do. I think we've data to strongly support it, but I don't know for certain that, in doing so, we're not creating a new set of difficulties. Similarly, we're providing the highest technology we possibly can to children. Still I think we're going in the right direction. I advocate, strongly support, and recommend to you that children be involved in their care as quickly as possible.

The whole foundation for this begins with appropriate positioning, and I can't leave an audience without talking about that. Everything—manipulation, communication, mobility, everything that we do for a child with a motor disability—begins with appropriate positioning. We say we won't let a psychologist, language pathologist, or educator at our patients because until they are appropriately positioned, they can't demonstrate their level of competence. Once they have functional control and the optimal ability to manipulate their world, then you can assess their strengths and needs—but only after you've appropriately positioned them.

I'll finish up here with just a couple of statements that you all know. "The role of parents must change from recipient of services to be an active participant in the decision-making process"—you know that. "The quality of the life of a child begins with the birth of his parents"—this is a statement we just can't forget. And I'll end up back with Sherri again, because that's where we started: a child, a family, and a community of resources. And if we put everything together, I would hope that we end up with a happy functioning child in a family within a community that understands what it's doing. I thank you very much.

12

Conclusion: Building on Existing Models to Expand Training Opportunities in the Future

Margo I. Peter
and
Rosalyn Benjamin Darling

This book represents an attempt to bridge the gap between professionals who provide medical services to children and parents who are responsible for their daily nurturing and caretaking, by promoting collaborative models of medical education. The ultimate goal is to improve the quality of medical care provided to children and their families. As the second author of this chapter pointed out in her introduction (Chapter 1), the disharmony of the traditionally disparate views of parents and professionals can be detrimental to the overall care of a child. Creating and implementing collaborative models of health care will ultimately enhance care and improve outcomes for children and their families.

In the past, medical education programs were based on the assumption that clinical competence was the overriding determinant of quality care. Physicians were trained to diagnose, treat, and cure, with little attention to the socioemotional needs of patients and their families. Over the years, we have learned more and more about the "art" of medicine. Clinical competence must be paired with and tempered by an understanding of human needs in order to be effective.

Traditionally, physicians were trained in a system of "professional dominance." They were taught to take control of the treatment situation and to be responsible for their actions. Patients generally accepted without question the physician's authority. Today, they are questioning more and more. Professional dominance is giving way to partnerships between doctors and patients.

Change is almost always difficult, and often threatening. No one feels comfortable when his or her expertise is perceived to be challenged. We must be careful in promoting new approaches to medical education. The clinical expertise of the physician is as valid today as it was in the past—*only its weight has changed.* The concept of partnership suggests that parental expertise can be equally valid.

When professional dominance is replaced by true collaboration, the burden of responsibility is shared. Families recognize that physicians and other professionals have special expertise as a result of their training and experience. On the other hand, professionals recognize that families understand their own routines, needs, and priorities better than anyone. To collaborate, the two must communicate. Physicians need to learn to ask the right questions and to listen to the answers. Until recently, few guideposts were available for professionals interested in working collaboratively with the families they served.

Now that the medical establishment is coming to recognize the validity of family-centered approaches, "nuts and bolts" methods must be made available to translate the philosophy into practice. Medical educators need curricula and models to emulate in designing new courses and programs for their students. We have tried, in this volume, to provide the resources these educators need to begin to teach medical professionals about working in partnership with families.

This book provides an excellent beginning point for individuals interested in improving the education systems responsible for training medical professionals. It provides a compendium of the various approaches being implemented across the country in medical schools, residency programs, and continuing medical education programs. While there are certainly other programs that remain unknown to the editors of this text, many—if not most—are represented or mentioned here. Sadly, such programs remain in the minority, and many physicians complete their training without acquiring the requisite skills for providing comprehensive family-centered care to children with special needs. Fortunately, there are programs like those described in this book to which we can turn to stimulate our creative thinking and obtain guidance as we develop and implement more such programs.

The wheels of change turn slowly, but turn they do. The movement toward equal, fair, and appropriate treatment for children with special needs has been nothing less than a civil rights movement. Children and families have unequivocally refused to sit at the back of the bus, and the system that serves them has improved accordingly. The process of change, however, is seldom easy. Growing pains are to be expected, especially as we contemplate changing a system with such long and venerated traditions. The important thing is to plot a course for positive change and navigate using the signposts left by earlier pioneers. The program designers described in this book are such pioneers. Several guiding principles emerge from their experience.

First, we much develop partnerships with parents and capitalize on their unique expertise as consumers and caretakers. Florene Poyadue points out in Chapter 2 that communication and cooperation are only the first steps toward collaboration. True collaboration involves working together toward a shared goal within a context of mutual trust and respect. Operationalized, this means that parents should have equal voice in program development and implementation. Parents like Sharon Spano (see Chapter 3) have a perspective that must be shared in any successful training program. Antoinette Eaton, past president of the American Academy of Pediatrics, has advocated for including parents as faculty members in universities and medical schools. Judy Lewis, Robert Greenstein, Nancy DiVenere, and Carl Cooley illustrate, in chapters 5, 6, and 7, ways in which this goal is being realized. Stanley Klein's Chapter 4 clearly describes a model for developing partnerships with parents in a clinical setting in order to improve clinical outcome.

Second, a consistent theme in all of the programs reviewed here is the importance of addressing physician attitudes in order to improve the quality of care they provide. Physician attitudes influence all levels of treatment, beginning with the initial diagnosis. Chapter 9 demonstrates how attitudes learned in a stigmatizing society can negatively affect the diagnostic process. In fact, the diagnostic interview is in many ways a microcosm of the treatment process. When handled appropriately, it includes most of the elements essential to optimal care for children with special health needs. Skills necessary for effective and appropriate response during the diagnostic process can be generalized to other treatment situations. This, combined with frequent complaints from parents regarding how diagnostic news is shared, makes the diagnostic process an essential content area to include in continuing medical education.

Third, one learns from this book the importance of tailoring programs to meet the unique needs of each setting. A variety of programs has been outlined, including those conducted in large and small group meetings, tertiary and home-based settings, and video and didactic formats. All have proven effective and each has unique merits. The variety represented here should encourage creativity and versatility in future endeavors.

Taken together, the models outlined represent a continuum of educational opportunities. In chapters 5 and 6, Judy Lewis, Robert Greenstein, and Nancy DiVenere present approaches for training medical students. In Chapter 7, Carl Cooley provides an overview of programs for pediatric residents. In chapters 8, 9, and 10, approaches used with continuing education audiences are reviewed by Rosalyn Darling, Francine Gallagher, Corinne Garland, Margo Peter, and Calvin Sia. Each is equally important because each impacts the clinician at a different stage in his or her professional development. Ideally, educational opportunities should be available at each of these junctures. The decision about where to begin is often a pragmatic one and depends largely on which of the three areas program organizers are in a position to influence. However, we must continue to advocate for the integration of this kind of training at all levels.

Fourth and finally, the importance of strong role models cannot be underestimated. Programs such as the ones mentioned here do not succeed without the dedicated efforts of physicians like Alfred Healy (see Chapter 11), Carl Cooley (see Chapter 7), Calvin Sia (see Chapter 8), and Robert Greenstein (see Chapter 5). Such individuals are leading the charge to promote optimal services for children and families, and it is their behavior that provides a living example for students to emulate.

There have always been physicians who have worked tirelessly to promote compassionate care for children. However, we are at a unique point in history, and a confluence of factors supports the role of these committed physicians as catalysts for systems change. Parents like Sharon Spano (see Chapter 3) have established their role in the system, and the call for family-centered care is being promoted (and funded) by federal regulatory agencies. This means that we have a prime opportunity to work together to assure that physicians are adequately prepared to fulfill their invaluable role as family allies. Fortunately, we can build on the foundation laid by the authors of these chapters.

Where will we go from here? Each state and local community will need to answer that question for itself. Certainly, medical schools, teaching hospitals, and community groups can begin immediately—if they have not already—to implement some of the suggested approaches described in this book or creative approaches of their own. However, statewide coordination of at least continuing education efforts is usually worthwhile.

State-level agencies such as the state chapter of the American Academy of Pediatrics, the Part H lead agency, and (if not the lead agency) the

Department of Health need to meet and develop strategies for providing training opportunities for physicians throughout the state. Although centralized conferences or workshops can be valuable, reaching *all* physicians usually means using local hospitals and other sites as well. "Train-the-trainers" and video-based models may be most effective for such widespread dissemination.

Regardless of the methods chosen, no effort will be successful unless representatives of two groups are included in the planning phase: community-based physicians, and families of children with special health needs. Practicing physicians are aware of their own time and interest limitations and know best how to reach their colleagues. Families need to be included to assure that no aspect of their perspective has been overlooked. As Sharon Spano's chapter (3) so movingly demonstrated, the family experience is best presented by families themselves.

Another suggestion—based on the 1992 conference that gave rise to this book—is the inclusion, in local training programs, of opportunities for open discussion among parents, physicians, and other professionals. Some of the best sessions at the conference were the small discussion groups that followed the general sessions. Both parents and professionals expressed satisfaction with the (rare) opportunity for a face-to-face exchange of views, feelings, and opinions. Such discussions could, of course, also be incorporated into medical school or residency curricula.

Finally, we will need to keep talking with one another. A wide range of professionals, including sociologists, psychologists, ethicists, child development specialists, therapists, educators, and others, must be included in these discussions along with physicians and families. As more education programs are developed and implemented, we must share our successes. The next conference may need to be longer than a day and a half. Eventually, specialized conferences on "family-centered care" or "parent–professional partnerships" should no longer be necessary at all, because these approaches will have become part of *mainstream* medicine. In the next century, family–professional collaboration should be the norm in pediatric, and perhaps all, medical care.

Resource List

BOOKS/PAMPHLETS/INFORMATION PACKETS

Available from the Association for the Care of Children's Health (7910 Woodmont Avenue, Suite 300, Bethesda, MD 20814-3015):

Family-Centered Care for Children with Special Health Care Needs (T. Shelton, E. Jeppson & B. Johnson, 1987).

Getting on Board: Training Activities to Promote the Practice of Family-Centered Care (L. Edelman, ed., 1991).

Physician Education Forum Report (National Center for Family-Centered Care, 1990).

Available from the Department of Maternal and Child Health, School of Hygiene and Public Health (Baltimore: The Johns Hopkins University):

Curriculum on Children with Special Health Care Needs and Their Families (H. Ireys & S. Gross, 1993).

Available from the Division of Developmental Disabilities, University Hospital School (Campus Stores, 208 G.S.B., University of Iowa, Iowa City, IA 52242):

Improving Health Care for Children with Chronic Conditions: Guidelines for Families (A. Healy & J. A. Lewis-Beck).

Available from The Evanston Hospital (The Infant Care Program, 2650 Ridge Avenue, Evanston, IL 60201):

A Hospital-Based, Multi-Disciplinary Approach to the Unexpected Delivery of an Infant with Down Syndrome (I. Cardone, S. Kraft, R. LaPata, P. Lawrence & I. Salafsky, eds., 1991).

Available from the National Maternal and Child Health Clearinghouse (8201 Greensboro Drive, Suite 600, McLean, VA 22102):

Family/Professional Collaboration for Children with Special Health Needs and Their Families (K. K. Bishop with J. Woll & P. Arango, 1993).

Available from the Parent Professional Partnership (Children's Hospital, 3705 Fifth Avenue, Pittsburgh, PA 15213-2538):

Our Future Lies in Working Together: Parents of Children with Developmental Delays Share Their Experiences with Professionals.

Available from Parents Helping Parents (535 Race Street, Suite 140, San Jose, CA 95126):

Better Ways (of breaking news to parents)—A Guide for Conducting a Workshop for Physicians (F. S. Poyadue).

Available from the University of Kansas Medical Center (3901 Rainbow Boulevard, Kansas City, KS 66160):

MEDLINKS Physician Folder (G. E. Holmes).

NEWSLETTERS

Available from the Center for Children with Chronic Illness and Disability (Box 721, University of Minnesota, 420 Delaware Street S.E., Minneapolis, MN 55455):

Springboard: The Newsletter of the Center for Children with Chronic Illness and Disability.

Children's Health Issues.

Available from the National Center for Family-Centered Care (7910 Woodmont Avenue, Suite 300, Bethesda, MD 20814):

Family-Centered Care Network.

VIDEOS

Available from The Institute for Families of Blind Children (P.O. Box 54700, Mailstop #111, Los Angeles, CA 90054-0700):

Breaking the News (physicians discuss their feelings), 1991.

Available from Beginnings (406 Main Street, Suite 201, Johnstown, PA 15901-1815):

Early Intervention: The Physician's Role in Referral (interviews with parents and physicians illustrating diagnosis and referral; also includes a twenty-five-page manual), 1990, 1993.

Available from Variety Preschoolers Workshop (47 Humphrey Drive, Syosset, NY 11791-4098, Attn: Barbara Sawicki):

The New Survivors (developed by parents of chronically ill children).

Available from Learner Managed Designs (2201 K West 25 Street, Lawrence, KS 66047):

Down Syndrome: A Parental Perspective.

MAGAZINE

Exceptional Parent (P.O. Box 3000, Dept. EP, Denville, NJ 07834).

Many other helpful books, articles, and chapters are included in the reference lists at the end of each chapter.

Index

Achievement, 4
Activism, 8–9
Acute illness, 54
Adapting and coping, 85–87
Adoption, 5
Affective neutrality, 6
Affectivity, 6
Alpert, J. S., 60, 63
Ambulatory Pediatric Association, 113
American Academy of Family Practice, 125
American Academy of Pediatrics, 124–125, 150–151, 152
American Board of Pediatrics, 150, 157
Anger, 67–68
Anomie, 6–7
Ascription, 4
Assertiveness training, 19
Assessment, 167–168
Association for Retarded Children, 174
Avoidance, 139

Baker, B. L., 55
Bernstein, L., 65–66
Bernstein, R. S., 65–66
Bijur, P. E., 112
Billings, J. A., 65
Biopsy, 36, 44
Birth, 140–141
Board certification, 111
Boyce, W. T., 112
Brazelton, T. B., 55
Breaking the News (Institute for Families of Blind Children), 60–61
Breastfeeding, 35
Brewer, E. J., Jr., 9
Buckman, R., 56, 61, 64–70
Building Parent/Professional Collaboration (Edelman, Greenland & Mills), 33–34

Cannon, Sheila, 2
Caplan, S., 52
Cardiac baby, 35
Caring for Infants and Toddlers project, 161–166
Case history, 63
Catheterization, 36
Causation, 86
Celiac disease, 48
Cerebral palsy, 65
Change, 22–23, 186
Child find, 166–167
Children, 177; caring for, 161–166,

173–183; miracle, 46–50; morbidity of, 123–128; roles of, 5–6; with special needs, 30
Cholden, L. S., 61
Christenson, Laurie, 67
Chronic conditions, 54, 80; impact on families, 83–85
Civil rights, 187
Clinical perspective, 5, 9
Clinical skills, 88–89
Collaboration, 17–27, 31, 161, 177; by-products of, 20; and early intervention, 152–153
Communication, 24, 175; challenge of, 51–72; with families, 41–43; lack of skills, 139–140
Community-based care, 126
Compliance, 54
Consumerism, 8
Continuing medical education (CME), 123–133, 156–158; and direct mail, 131–132; Hawaiian, 125; heart and soul of, 127; large group/grand rounds format, 129–131; train-the-trainers model, 128–129
Cooley, Carl W., 2, 162
Coordinated care, 126–127
"Creating Family–Professional Partnerships," 2
Creative problem solving, 26
Crisp, R., 77
Cruickshank, W. M., 58
Cytochrome C Oxidase Deficiency, 40–42, 44, 49

Darling, R. B., 1, 3, 5
Dartmouth–Hitchcock Medical Center, 115–116
Davis, F., 141
Deafness, 42
Delivering difficult news, 60–63
Denial, 67–68
Depression, 68
Desire to work together, 24–25
Developmental screening methods, 155
Diagnosis, 1, 50; and referrals, 135–147
Diagnostic news, 17, 60–70
Difference, 24
Diffuseness, 5–6
Direct mail, 131–132
Disability, adapting to, 85–87
Doctor–patient relationship, 87
Down syndrome, 19, 77, 183

Early intervention: obstacles to, 135–147; physicians' needs for information about, 149–166
Early Intervention: The Physician's Role in Referral (1990), 143
Echocardiogram, 36
Education for All Handicapped Children Act, 8
Education of the Handicapped Act (EHA), 149
Ego: fragile, 21; healthy, 26
Emerson, D. L., 68
Empathy, 59
Entitlement, 150
Euphemisms, 64, 140
Evaluation design, 81–82
Exceptional Parent magazine, 9, 69
Expectant mother, 23
Expectations, 38–41
Eyeglasses, 19

Failure, 138–139
Families, 175–176; building partnerships with, 32–46; communication with, 41–43; hope for, 46–50; impact of chronic illness on, 83–85; recruitment and orientation of, 102–103
Family-centered care, 30–32, 127–128
Family–physician interaction, 2–10
Family studies, 118
Fathers, 56–57
Fear, 21
Fragile egos, 21
Francis, V., 7
Freidson, E., 3, 6–7
Freud, S., 68
Future, 176
Future of Pediatric Education (American Academy of Pediatrics), 109

Gastrostomy, 87
Gatekeepers, 147
Genetic counseling, 179
Gething, L., 77

Getting to Yes: Negotiating Agreement without Giving In (Fisher et al.), 44
Goffman, E., 138
Golden, S., 72
Grant, J. O., 58
Green, M., 123
Greenspan, S. I., 55
Guralnick, M. J., 114, 136, 152, 158

Haggerty, R. J., 123
Handicapped Infants and Toddlers Program (Part H), 149–150, 152, 158–160
Haug, M. R., 8, 140
Healy, A., 136
Heiser, K. E., 136
Henkind, P., 65
Hinting, 140
Holden, R. H., 141
Home visits, 105–106
Honesty, 25
Hope, 46–50
How to Break Bad News (Buckman), 64
Hutchins, V. L., 9
Hyshimoto's disease, 48

Immunization, 11
Imperfection, 30
Individual Education Plan (IEP), 18
Individuality, 87–88
Individuals with Disabilities Education Act (IDEA), 8, 149
Information dosages, 68–69, 71
Introduction to Clinical Medicine (ICM-A), 78–81, 95–99; chronic conditions, 80; conclusions, 99; continuing impact, 93–95; course objectives of, 96–97; evaluation design of, 81–82; genetics program, 81, 97–98; patient-family response to, 90–93; results of, 82–98
Introductory lecture, 104–105
Ireys, H. T., 10

Journal of Pediatrics, 108

Kohrt, Alan, 2
Koop, C. Everett, 20, 126
Kopp, Sheldon, 21
Korsch, B. M., 7, 54–55

Labor, 20, 23
Lack of knowledge, 137
Lamaze classes, 29
Language, understandable, 60
Large group/grand rounds format, 129–131
Lavin, B., 8, 140
Leadership, 163–164
Leukemia, 178
Lipton, H. L., 139
Lorch, S. C., 117

McPherson, M., 9
Magrab, P. R., 9
Medical education, 101–108; continuing, 123–133
Medical Education Project, 101–108
Medical home, 124, 136
Mendosa, Jeanne, 23–24
Mercer, J. R., 5
Michigan State University, 117–118
Mitochondrial disorders, 44
Models, 71; development of, 142; physician education, 2; train-the-trainers, 128–129
Morbidity, new, 123–128
Morris, M. J., 7
Morse, W. C., 58
Mother, expectant, 23
Mourning, 61, 65, 85
Murphee, A. Linn, 62
Mutual respect, 24, 33–37
Mystification, 140

Negative socialization, 137–138
Negrete, V., 55
Nelson, R. P., 10
Neonatal Intensive Care Unit, 156
Neurosis, 21–22
Noncompliance, 7
Nonreferral, 136–141
Normal living patterns, 176
Nutrition, 43

Pain, 31
Parent activism, 8–9
Parental distress, 64–67

Parenthood, 3
Parent–professional collaboration, 17–27
Parents: attitudes of, 86–87; attitudes toward, 52–55; as educators, 101–108; as experts, 54; label of, 20; observations by, 60; partnerships with, 187; reticence of, 7; role of, 3–4, 183
Parent to Parent of Vermont, 102–103
Parsons, T., 3
Particularism, 4–5
Partnership, 32–46, 58–60
Passing the buck, 140
Paternalism, 140–141
Patient, individuality of, 87–88
Patient-as-teacher experience, 89–90
"Patient education information," 51
Patient/family response, 90–93
Pediatricians' Early Intervention Questionnaire, 154–155
Pediatrics, 109–119; and the new morbidity, 125–132; and reliable allies, 110–111; residency training, 111–118; survey on early intervention, 152–161; type of practice, 153–154
Perfection, tyranny of, 21
Peter, M. I., 53–54, 62
Phillips, Carol, 103
Physician education, 2, 101–108
Physicians: attitudes of, 187; competencies required by, 181; confidence in, 8; and early intervention, 149–166; as gatekeepers, 147; new roles for, 161–166
Pieper, Betty, 1, 5
Planning, 58
Poetry, 27
Points of view, 26
"Pop psychology," 52–53
Powers, J. T., 136
Preconceptional counseling, 178
Pregnancies, high-risk, 179
Prejudices, 53
Preliminary evaluation, 144–146
Presentation, 63–64
Prevention, 181–182
Primary care, 1, 9, 175
Primary care physicians (PMDs), 125; and community-based care, 126; and coordinated care, 126–127; and family-centered care, 127–128
Professional dominance, 6–7
Professionals: changing attitudes of, 9–10; interaction with, 1; number of, 57–58; rich, heartless, 20–21; roles of, 3–8; suggestions for, 37, 40–41
Prognosis, uncertainty of, 141
Project Bridge, 151
Project evaluation and significance, 164–165
Providers, 31
Psychosocial concerns, 6

Quality of life, 43, 85–86

Referrals, 135, 155–156
Reliable allies, 110–111
Religion, 86
Residency training, 111–114; innovations in, 114–118
Respect, 24, 33–37
Respite care, 115
Richardson, S. A., 5
Roles, 188; of children, 5–6; clarification of, 38–41; new, for physicians, 161–166; of parents, 3–4, 183; of professionals, 3–8
Rousso, H., 70

Scott, F. G., 152–161, 165
Self-esteem, 55
Services, 176, 180
Setting, 55–56
Sharp, M. C., 117
Shock, 94
Shonkoff, J., 151
Sia, C., 53–54, 62
Socialization, 3; lack of, 137–138
Social system perspective, 5
Solving problems, 43–46
Specificity, 5–6
Spina bifida, 3
Spina Bifida Association of America, 3
Stacey, M., 6
St. Christopher's Children's Hospital, 116–117
Step-by-step presentation, 63–64
Stevens, Trudy, 23–24

Stifler, D., 101, 105
Stimson, G., 7
Stoeckle, J. D., 65
Stress of clinical care, 52
Strong, P. M., 7
Student logs, 82–90
Students: follow-up lecture for, 106; impact on, 93–95; introductory lecture for, 104–105; parents as educators of, 101–108
Support groups, 7, 69–70
Surgery, 44–45
Survey of Pediatricians, 152–161
Svarstad, B. L., 139
Swartz, D., 101, 104–105, 107

Task Force on Education in Developmental Pediatrics, 151
Touching, 68
Training, 70–71, 162–163; in the future, 185–189
Train-the-trainer approach, 128–129
Tremors, 43

Universalism, 4–5
University of Maryland, 116
University of North Carolina, 117

Validation, 72

Wabrek, A. J., 62, 66
Wachtel, R. C., 116
Webb, B., 7
Wender, E. H., 112
Wenger, M., 152
Witt, J. E., 55
Wittenberg, S. M., 60, 63
Wolraich, M. L., 3
Worldviews, 2–7
Wright, B. A., 77
Wright, Kenneth W., 61
Writing skills, 71
Written reports, 70

About the Editors and Contributors

W. CARL COOLEY, M.D., is a Developmental Pediatrician and is Associate Director of Clinical Services at the Dartmouth Center for Genetics and Child Development in Lebanon, New Hampshire. He is medical director of a statewide network of outreach programs for children with special health care needs. His research interests focus on methods of enhancing the capacity of communities to serve children with special health needs and their families, family adaptations to having a child with special needs, and issues of individuals with Down syndrome. Dr. Cooley's background includes service as a primary pediatrician in a small New Hampshire community. He is also the father of a child with a disability.

Mailing Address: W. Carl Cooley, M.D., Associate Director for Clinical Services, Assistant Professor of Pediatrics, Dartmouth Center for Genetics and Child Development, Dartmouth Hitchcock Medical Center, Lebanon, NH 03756.

ROSALYN BENJAMIN DARLING, Ph.D., is Assistant Professor of Sociology at Indiana University of Pennsylvania. For the past fifteen years she was Executive Director of Beginnings Early Intervention Services of Cambria County, Incorporated, and Adjunct Assistant Professor of Sociology at the University of Pittsburgh at Johnstown. Dr. Darling, who is a medical sociologist, is the author of four books and many articles and chapters about children with disabilities and their families. She is currently working on a fifth book on family methods in early intervention, to be

published by Pro-Ed next year. Dr. Darling has also served on several committees of Pennsylvania's Interagency Coordinating Council for Early Intervention. Her professional interests include family–professional interaction and sociological aspects of disability.
Mailing Address: Rosalyn B. Darling, Ph.D., Department of Sociology, Keith Hall, Indiana University of Pennsylvania, Indiana, PA 15705-1087.

NANCY J. DIVENERE is the Director of Parent to Parent of Vermont, a nationally recognized peer support and information network for families whose children have a chronic illness or disability. She has extensive experience designing and implementing training projects, including the Medical Education Project. Ms. DiVenere is the parent of three children, the youngest of whom has special health and educational needs.
Mailing Address: Nancy DiVenere, Director, Parent to Parent of Vermont, 1 Main Street, #69 Champlain Mill, Winooski, VT 05404.

FRANCINE GORTLER GALLAGHER, M.Ed., is the Project Coordinator for Child Development Resources' "Caring for Infants and Toddlers with Disabilities: New Roles for Physicians" inservice training project. Ms. Gallagher, in her role as Part H Project Assistant, has served as a staff member of the Virginia Interagency Coordinating Council (VICC). She was also the staff person for VICC's Child Find and Public Awareness committees. She has experience in early intervention service delivery and in planning and implementing training for early intervention professionals serving infants and toddlers with disabilities.
Mailing Address: Francine Gortler Gallagher, M.Ed., Project Coordinator, Child Development Resources, P.O. Box 299, Lightfoot, VA 23090-0299.

CORINNE W. GARLAND, M.Ed., is the Executive Director of Child Development Resources in Lightfoot, Virginia. Ms. Garland is experienced in the administration of early intervention services in the public, private, and university sectors. She has been involved in the development and implementation of inservice training and technical assistance for early intervention providers, with emphasis on the transdisciplinary approach. She has served as President of the International Division of Early Childhood of the Council for Exceptional Children, and is currently the Division's Governor. She served a three-year term as a governor's appointee to the Virginia Interagency Coordinating Council (VICC) and as Chair of its Service Delivery Committee.
Mailing Address: Corinne W. Garland, M.Ed., Executive Director, Child Development Resources, P.O. Box 299, Lightfoot, VA 23090-0299.

ROBERT M. GREENSTEIN, M.D., is Professor of Pediatrics and Director of the Division of Human Genetics at the University of Connecticut School of Medicine. He joined the Department of Pediatrics in 1969 following a fellowship in birth defects and genetics at Stanford University Medical School. Since that time, he has continuously provided programs of service and research for children with disabilities and their families. He has also provided continuing education programs for a wide variety of professionals in the fields of health care, education, and public health. Dr. Greenstein is on the Board of Directors of the Connecticut Down Syndrome Congress and is a previous Chair of the Governor's Council on Mental Retardation for the State of Connecticut.
Mailing Address: Robert M. Greenstein, M.D., Professor, Department of Pediatrics, MC-6310, The School of Medicine of the University of Connecticut Health Center, Farmington, CT 06030.

ALFRED HEALY, M.D., is Professor of Pediatrics and Director of the Division of Developmental Disabilities in the College of Medicine, as well as Professor of Curriculum and Instruction in the College of Education, at the University of Iowa. He has served as a member of the faculty at the university for the past twenty-eight years and as Director of the University Hospital School since 1977. His major interests are in developing supports for children with disabilities and their families, and in increasing the involvement of pediatricians in their care. He has served as president of a number of professional organizations, as well as Chair of the American Academy of Pediatrics National Committee on Children with Disabilities.
Mailing Address: Alfred Healy, M.D., Director, Iowa University Affiliated Program, University Hospital School, University of Iowa, Iowa City, IA 52242.

STANLEY D. KLEIN, Ph.D., is Co-founder and Publisher of *Exceptional Parent* magazine. He is also Professor of Psychology and Director of the Counseling Service at the New England College of Optometry in Boston. Dr. Klein also serves as a Research Associate in Medicine (General Pediatrics) at Children's Hospital in Boston, where he teaches pediatricians about working with the parents of children with disabilities. He also teaches at Tufts/New England Medical Center, Department of Rehabilitation Medicine. Dr. Klein is the author of *Psychological Testing of Children: A Consumer's Guide* (1975) and co-editor of *The Disabled Child and the Family: An Exceptional Parent Reader* (1985) and *It Isn't Fair! Siblings of Children with Disabilities* (1993).

Mailing Address: Stanley D. Klein, Ph.D., Exceptional Parent, 209 Harvard Street, Brookline, MA 02146-5005.

JUDY LEWIS, M.Phil., is the Director of Community Based Education and Associate Professor in the Department of Community Medicine at the University of Connecticut School of Medicine. She received her professional training in medical sociology at Yale University and has been on the faculty at the University of Connecticut since 1973. Ms. Lewis has worked with community programs in the greater Hartford area to broaden medical and public health education. She chairs the Primary Care Clerkship and works with medical and M.P.H. students on community health projects in the United States and other countries. Her primary areas of interest are medical education and maternal and child health.
Mailing Address: Judy Lewis, M.Phil., Associate Professor, Department of Community Medicine and Health Care, University of Connecticut Health Center, Farmington, CT 06030-1910.

MERLE MCPHERSON, M.D., M.P.H., is currently Director of the Division of Services for Children with Special Health Needs of the U.S. Bureau of Maternal and Child Health. She received her medical degree from the University of Saskatchewan in Canada in 1959 and holds a Master of Public Health degree from the Johns Hopkins School of Public Health. Dr. McPherson is a fellow of the American Board of Preventive Medicine and of the American Board of Pediatrics and has worked in pediatric clinical settings at the local, state, and international levels. She has had administrative responsibility for the Title V Crippled Children's Program, for primary pediatric care in the District of Columbia, and for the Title V Maternal and Child Health Program and Family Health Services in the State of Hawaii. Dr. McPherson has held various positions in the Maternal and Child Health program at the federal level since 1976 and is the recipient of numerous honors and awards.
Mailing Address: Merle McPherson, M.D., M.P.H., Director, Division of Services for Children with Special Health Needs, Maternal and Child Health Bureau, Parklawn Building, Room 948-5600, Fishers Lane, Rockville, MD 20857.

MARGO I. PETER, M.Ed., was the Project Director of the Medical Home Project of the Hawaii Medical Association. She has worked with children and families for sixteen years in a variety of capacities including as a Special Educator, School Psychologist, and Infant Development Specialist. Through the Medical Home Project, she worked to enhance physician involvement in the care of children with special needs.

Mailing Address: Margo I. Peter, M.Ed., 45-020 A Malulani Street, Kaneohe, HI 96744.

FLORENE STEWART POYADUE, R.N., M.A., M.F.C.C., B.V.E., is the Chief Executive Officer of Parents Helping Parents (PHP) in San Jose, California—an organization she founded along with other parents of children with special needs. PHP is now the National Center on Parent Directed Family Resource Centers. Ms. Poyadue graduated magna cum laude from St. Mary's Infirmary School of Nursing. She received her Bachelor of Vocational Education degree from San Jose State University, and her Master's degree in counseling, as well as an honorary doctorate in public service, from Santa Clara University. Ms. Poyadue is the mother of four children, one of whom has Down syndrome. An American of African heritage, she is very much involved in issues of cultural competence and human relations.
Mailing Address: Florene Stewart Poyadue, PHP, Suite 140, 535 Race Street, San Jose, CA 95126.

CALVIN C. J. SIA, M.D., F.A.A.P., has been in primary care pediatric practice since 1958 in Honolulu, Hawaii. He is currently the Chair of the American Medical Association Section Council on Pediatrics and Delegate for the American Academy of Pediatrics in the AMA House. He has been President of the Hawaii Medical Association, Hawaii Chapter of the American Academy of Pediatrics, and is Clinical Professor of Pediatrics at the University of Hawaii School of Medicine. Dr. Sia is a board member of the American Board of Pediatrics and a past member of the National Advisory Council on Child Health and Human Development of the National Institutes of Health. He is a child advocate with interests in community pediatrics, beginning with Head Start, school health, special education, and child abuse and neglect, with recent initiatives in prevention and early intervention. Dr. Sia recently received the Third C. Henry Kempe Award, the Abraham Jacobi Award of the American Medical Association and the American Academy of Pediatrics, and an Honorary Doctorate of Humane Letters from the University of Hawaii.
Mailing Address: Calvin C. J. Sia, M.D., 1350 S. King Street, Suite 300, Honolulu, HI 96814.

SHARON L. SPANO is a Family Advocate and Trainer who has done extensive work relating to early intervention services for infants and toddlers. As the mother of a child with special needs, she has a strong commitment to the spirit and philosophy of Part H of Public Law 99-457 and

the principles of family-centered care. Her experience and commitment have resulted in the coordination, development, and implementation of the Physicians' Training Project in Florida and extensive training on the philosophical framework of family-centered care and Florida's Family Support Plan. She continues to work in these areas as a consultant with Family Systems Design Associates.
Mailing Address: Sharon L. Spano, Family Systems Design Associates, 110 Alafaya Woods Boulevard, Suite B, Oviedo, FL 32765.

BONNIE STRICKLAND, Ph.D., is a Public Health Analyst in the U.S. Bureau of Maternal and Child Health. Her background is in special education, and she previously was an Associate Professor at Cleveland State University and Director of Early Childhood Programs at the Family Child Learning Center of Akron, Ohio. She has taught at the University of North Carolina at Chapel Hill and served as a Special Education Director. Her publications include three books and various articles and chapters.
Mailing Address: Bonnie Strickland, Ph.D., Public Health Analyst, Bureau of Maternal and Child Health, Room 18A-20, Parklawn Building, 5600 Fishers Lane, Rockville, MD 20857.

ISBN 0-86569-226-2
90000>
EAN
9 780865 692268
HARDCOVER BAR CODE